PROSTATECTOMY

Edited by **Tsvetin Genadiev**

Prostatectomy
http://dx.doi.org/10.5772/intechopen.73923
Edited by Tsvetin Genadiev

Contributors

Elisabeth Eppard, Tanya Stoyanova, Meghan Rice, Yukio Naya, Kazuhiro Araki, Wai Hee Steve Chan, Chi Fai Kan, Churk Fai Trevor Li, Michael Whalen, Yusuf İlker Comez, Tsvetin Trifonov Genadiev

First published in London, United Kingdom, 2019 by IntechOpen
IntechOpen is the global imprint of INTECHOPEN LIMITED, registered in England and Wales, registration number: 11086078, The Shard, 25th floor, 32 London Bridge Street
London, SE19SG – United Kingdom
Printed in Croatia

British Library Cataloguing-in-Publication Data
A catalogue record for this book is available from the British Library

Additional hard and PDF copies can be obtained from orders@intechopen.com

Prostatectomy, Edited by Tsvetin Genadiev
p. cm.
Print ISBN 978-1-83880-684-2
Online ISBN 978-1-83880-685-9
eBook (PDF) ISBN 978-1-83880-686-6

For EU product safety concerns:
IN TECH d.o.o., Prolaz Marije Krucifikse Kozulić 3, 51000 Rijeka, Croatia,
info@intechopen.com or visit our website at intechopen.com.

Meet the editor

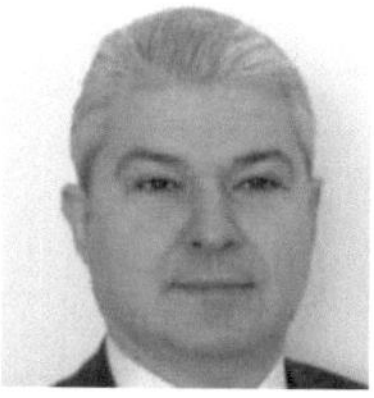

Associate Professor Tsvetin Genadiev graduated from the Medical University of Sofia, Bulgaria. He has a PhD in Urology from the same university and became Associate Professor of Urology in the Faculty of Medicine of Sofia University, St. Kliment Ohridski. Doctor Genadiev introduced and developed laparoscopy in Bulgarian urology and established this method in the practice. He is a researcher in the field of prostate gland and initiator and founder of the Prostate Center in Vita Hospital, Sofia, Bulgaria. Today, he is a consultant urologist in this hospital.

Contents

Preface

It is a great honor for me to have been chosen and invited to be the editor of this book. It inspired me to work with various colleagues from around the world on an ongoing research and development topic in medicine—the prostate gland. The book presents some new challenges and hypotheses in the field of contemporary diagnosis of prostate cancer.

The reader will also discover unpublished methods and hypotheses for one of the most commonly performed surgical techniques in urology—the technique of prostatectomy. The concept of early diagnosis of prostate cancer, minimally invasive surgical treatment, and rapid recovery methods are on track to alter prostate urology.

The editing of this book and its final publication were possible due to the active and dedicated cooperation of the publishing management team and especially of Mr. Julian Virag, for which I express my gratitude.

Associate Prof. Tsvetin Genadiev
Department of Urology
Vita Hospital
Sofia, Bulgaria

Section 1

Introduction to Prostatectomy - Challenges in the Past and Present

Chapter 1

Introductory Chapter: Prostatectomy - Challenge in the Past and Today

Tsvetin Trifonov Genadiev

Additional information is available at the end of the chapter

http://dx.doi.org/10.5772/intechopen.81804

1. Prostate and prostate surgery through the centuries

This short historical review shows the meaning of the prostate and the main points in the development of prostatectomy techniques through the centuries. The historical documents reveal the contribution of a large number of names of distinguished doctors and scholars from the ancient centuries to the present day. It is difficult to present this contribution in detail within an article, but it is possible to identify the main points of prostate surgery and their significance these days.

Documents show that the term "prostate" has an ancient origin. The term has been described by ancient anatomists but has become important for urine retention around the middle of the sixteenth century. A century later, metal catheters and tools for urinating through the prostate began to be used.

At the end of the seventeenth and the beginning of the eighteenth century, the urinary stone surgery marked a turbulent development through perineal access to the urethra and bladder. After the profound anatomical studies of the peritoneum by the Douglas brothers, it is clear that the peritoneum can be preserved and separated from the bladder during surgery. John Douglas performed a suprapubic surgery for bladder stones, which he calls as high operation. It replaces the perineal surgery for a short time. This finding can be considered the basis of suprapubic urological surgery. These two surgical techniques—perineal and suprapubic—become the basis of modern prostate surgery.

The introduction of anaesthesia and aseptic treatment began the violent development in urological surgery in the second half and the end of the nineteenth century. A number of remarkable surgeons perform for the first time operations to remove bladder stones and prostate parts through suprapubic access. A new problem faces them—the bladder healing that remains open after surgery. Surgical progress achieves surgery with primary bladder closure. The enucleation of the whole prostate gland through the operator's finger becomes a key point in this surgery. It has been used to treat enlarged prostate and urine retention. Operative techniques become a challenge for surgeons. Conflicts between remarkable surgeons for pioneering in surgical techniques arise. At that time, these operations were performed to treat urinary retention of the enlarged prostate, and the cancer had not yet been studied. The first described histological case of prostate cancer dates back to the middle of the nineteenth century. The problem is developing vigorously in the early twentieth century with the development and practice. New challenges are found in prostate surgeons—cancer removal. The urologists had hardly achieved successful surgical technique for adenoma and had to experience the new challenge of radical prostatectomy.

In the first half of the twentieth century, the main goal of prostate surgery remains the low mortality and successfully completed surgery, but achieving these goals does not stop the progression of prostatectomy. In addition to open techniques, through perineal, suprapubic, retropubic, inguinal, transcoccigeal, ischiorectal access, transurethral surgery is also widely used in practice. It also provides a combined operation—suprapubic access with transurethral one for good haemostasis.

The development of early diagnosis of prostate cancer sets new goals for urologists—achieving quality of surgery and quality of life for the patient. The investigation of pelvic anatomy leads to the discovery of a new prostatectomy—a nerve-sparing radical prostatectomy. This discovery becomes the basis of all modern surgical techniques for the treatment of prostate cancer. The refinement and standardisation of open surgery for prostate adenoma and prostate carcinoma seem to satisfy the aspirations of modern twentieth century surgery. At the end of this period, the challenge of laparoscopic technique began in various areas of surgery. This technique sets new targets for surgeons—surgery without harm to the patient—a basic law in surgery.

The love of urology and medical dedication to the patient justify this considerable progress of prostatectomy. Today, the technology revolution, along with classical experience, rewarded the surgeon with the introduction of the robotic operation. It protects the surgeon's health and awaits his full dedication to the patient. Nevertheless, the challenges of prostatectomy do not stop. New and new methods based on laparoscopy and transurethral surgery continue to be performed.

2. Brief introduction to the chapters

2.1. Section prostate diagnosis

The first chapter of this section presents the novel smart method for prostate diagnosis based on the spectroscopy. The method is expected to diagnose the effect of prostate cancer treatment and to provide accurate and personalised patient monitoring. This will improve the healing tactics of each patient.

The second chapter presents and discusses the different invasive and noninvasive biomarkers for prostate cancer early diagnosis and good therapy selection. The genetic diagnosis for prostate cancer is the near future of this field.

http://dx.doi.org/10.5772/intechopen.81804

The last chapter presents a new diagnostic method for positron emission scanning the prostate cancer, local or metastatic disease, using scandium. This pharmaceutic has a longer half-life than the gallium and has advantages in this diagnostic method.

2.2. Section prostatectomy operative techniques

This section introduces new methods for simple and radical prostatectomy. The authors describe the methods and present their results. It is interesting to see the different key points of some classical urological operative techniques and their new applications.

2.3. Section prostatectomy recovery and quality of life

The goal of modern radical prostatectomy is not only to be a healing method for prostate cancer but also to achieve good functional outcomes for the quality of life of the patient. This section presents a very extensive and in-depth scientific work on the topic of patient recovery after radical prostatectomy.

3. Conclusion

This book is a modest document of contemporary efforts and challenges in the diagnosis and treatment of a significant area of modern medicine—the prostate. There is hardly any other part of urology that has caused such an endless and meaningful century-old progression comparable to that of the prostate gland surgery.

We hope the reader will find answers to his questions and a spark of new challenges to prostatectomy!

Author details

Tsvetin Trifonov Genadiev

Address all correspondence to: genadievi@abv.bg

Department of Urology, Vita Hospital, Sofia, Bulgaria

Section 2

Prostate Diagnosis - Biomarkers

Chapter 2

Biomarkers for Diagnosis and Prognosis of Prostate Cancer

Meghan A. Rice and Tanya Stoyanova

Additional information is available at the end of the chapter

http://dx.doi.org/10.5772/intechopen.79726

Abstract

Since its discovery, elevated prostate-specific antigen (PSA) has been the measurement to indicate possibility of prostate cancer, as well as biochemical recurrence following treatment. Although PSA has led to decrease in prostate cancer–related mortalities, PSA is a nonspecific prostate cancer biomarker reflective of other prostate-related conditions such as benign prostatic hyperplasia (BPH), resulting in a high false-positive rate. This has led to overtreatment of men with clinically insignificant disease. While most prostate cancer patients have slowly progressive disease and should be treated conservatively, roughly 10% of patients will progress to have metastatic disease, of which the majority of prostate cancer deaths can be attributed. Stratifying these patients based on prognosis so that they may benefit from aggressive treatment is critical to their survival. Biomarkers for prostate cancer diagnosis and subsequent prognostic screening have significantly advanced this field. Here, we review some of the current blood, tissue, and urine biomarker tools used to measure an array of molecules including DNA, RNA, protein, or even epigenetic modifications. Utilizing the technologies described here, as well as looking to the future, correct early identification of prostate cancer with powerful prognostic value is much closer than ever before.

Keywords: prostate cancer, biomarker, early detection, prognosis, risk stratification

1. Introduction

Prostate cancer remains the most commonly diagnosed cancer in men in the United States with over 200,000 new cases detected annually [1]. Gleason grade of prostate cancer, developed by Dr. Donald Gleason in the 1960s, remains the most prognostic indicator of prostate cancer to date. Gleason grade ranges from 1 (normal) to 5 (most abnormal) and is assigned based on the histology of prostate tissues from biopsies. The Gleason score ranges from 2 to 10 and is the sum of the two most common Gleason grades. However, assessing Gleason grade requires invasive tissue biopsies. Less than one-third of men tested for prostate cancer through biopsy are diagnosed with cancer by histological analysis. Meanwhile a negative biopsy does little to reassure patients and clinicians of negative cancer status. This leads to a large number of patients undergoing painful initial biopsy procedures that may ultimately be repeated due to uncertainty of diagnosis [2]. Prostate cancer biopsies are a painful and invasive procedure, with the chance of complications including bleeding and infection [3–5].

Of those patients with positive diagnoses, roughly 10% will progress to metastatic prostate cancer, resulting in about 30,000 deaths annually in the United States. It is obvious that these patients should receive aggressive treatment at the earliest sign of disease. However there is concern as to over-diagnosis and over-treatment of indolent prostate cancer [6], resulting in some cases of high risk prostate cancer being treated conservatively with active surveillance, or first step intervention with radiation or radical prostatectomy. It is imperative to the respective disparate patient populations to receive the most accurate, timely, prognostic diagnosis.

The national cancer institute (NCI) dictionary of cancer terms defines biomarker as a "biological molecule found in blood, other body fluids, or tissues that is a sign of a normal or abnormal process, or a condition or disease." Advancements in the field of biomarker discovery have shaped the way medicine is performed and patients are diagnosed [7]. Biomarkers are used throughout the scope of clinical progression from early detection and diagnosis through clinical endpoint determinations.

Ideal biomarkers should have high sensitivity and specificity. That is, the power to correctly identify a high proportion of true cases, or those that will experience an event - in this case, developing prostate cancer. A biomarker should also have high specificity, correctly identifying patients who are truly negative for harboring prostate cancer. Typically, a balance is met between specificity and sensitivity. These results are presented as receiver operating characteristic (ROC) curves which are a visual means to describe the statistical ability of a model to correctly classify cases from non-cases [8]. Complete random distribution creates an "area under the curve" or AUC value of 0.50, graphed as a straight slope line, while the value from a perfect prediction model would be 1.0. A reliable prediction model therefore should have an AUC value nearing 1.0.

Here we will discuss the scope of biomarkers currently used for prostate cancer diagnosis, as well as prognosis to aid in disease monitoring and treatment oriented decision-making. Prostate cancer biomarkers are currently among three categories: blood, tissue or urine based biomarkers.

2. Blood-based biomarkers

An ideal biomarker screen is non-invasive. Blood collection is considered a minimally invasive technique with quick turnaround time that is also indicative of real-time alterations and disease states in the body, while robust or stable enough for findings to be reproducible across clinics. For prostate cancer as with many other diseases, the use of blood to monitor disease progression was the first and hallmark analysis performed to detect the disease.

In recent years, the phrase "liquid biopsy" has been coined, expanding a simple blood draw into an extensive cancer screen, testing for circulating tumor cells or circulating tumor free DNA in the blood. These tests have shown great promise in detecting cancer at early stages across a wide array of malignancies including prostate cancer [9].

Today, we continue to use blood based screens as means to detect prostate cancer, inform patients and clinicians on necessity of treatment, as well as to plan and monitor treatment response.

2.1. Prostate-specific antigen

The discovery of prostate and prostatic fluid associated antigens, most notably prostate-specific antigen (PSA) occurred in 1970 by Richard Ablin [10]. PSA is a glycoprotein produced by human kallikrein-3 (hK3), a member of a class of highly homologous serine proteases, the tissue kallikreins. PSA is normally produced by the epithelial cells of the prostate gland and secreted into the lumen to aid in liquefaction of semen ejaculate. However, other pathological conditions in the prostate, such as benign prostatic hyperplasia (BPH) or prostatitis can elevate the serum PSA levels, resulting in a "false positive" PSA test. PSA concentration in blood has been heavily explored for detection of prostate cancer, as well as treatment response and progression free survival monitoring thereof.

The number of diagnosed prostate cancer cases surged with the implementation of PSA screening tests, peaking at around the time of its approval by the United Stated Food and Drug Administration (FDA) in 1994 for prostate cancer detection. While PSA is prostate specific, it is not, however, specific to cancer, being additionally increased in the aforementioned benign prostate conditions. Since its discovery, PSA has been extensively studied in randomized clinical trials as a screening test for prostate cancer. Despite this discovery, prostate cancer remains the most commonly diagnosed non-cutaneous cancer in men in the United States, with solid tumor-associated deaths only second to lung cancer [1]. In addition to poor cancer specificity, PSA also has low sensitivity. Reported in the prostate cancer prevention trial (PCPT) 15% of men with PSA 0–4 ng/ml have prostate cancer, 15% of those are high Gleason score [11, 12].

Ultimately, implementation of PSA as a screening tool led to an over-diagnosis and subsequent over-treatment of low-risk disease. Perspective studies indicated up to 10% of patients who received curative therapy by either radical prostatectomy or radiation were over-treated [13]. In 2012 The United States Preventative Services Task Force (USPSTF) recommended against PSA based screening for prostate cancer [14]. This recommendation has recently been amended to suggest PSA may be used specifically in men 55–69 on a case-by-case basis with informed patient consent regarding potential harms of screening. In all, the usefulness of PSA will continue to persist especially in disease monitoring, but recent advances lose faith in PSA alone as a diagnostic tool. In-depth analysis of PSA has revealed several molecular variations and functions of PSA which may prove to be more specific to cancerous tissues.

2.1.1. Free vs. bound PSA

PSA is typically observed complexed to protease inhibitors such as alpha 1-antichymotrypsin (ACT) or alpha 2-macroglobulin, known as bound PSA [15, 16]. Discovered in the 1990s, a higher ratio of free PSA, that is, not bound to protease inhibitors and considered inactive, is associated with increased likelihood of BPH rather than cancer [15, 17–19]. Specific assays have also been developed to measure bound PSA (complexed-PSA), which is usually PSA-ACT and is elevated in cancer [20]. A percentage free PSA (free PSA/total PSA) can be calculated, and is typically lower in men with prostate cancer [21], where early studies linked <25% free PSA to detection of prostate cancer with a sensitivity of 95% [22]. However, follow-up analyses have had less promising results likely due to the relative instability of free or uncomplexed PSA compared to bound, making this an unreliable clinical parameter for patient diagnosis [23, 24].

2.1.2. Proenzyme PSA (proPSA)

Free PSA can be found in three different forms; proenzyme PSA (proPSA), benign PSA (BPSA) and intact PSA. proPSA is found increased in patients with prostate cancer [25, 26]. Several isoforms exist of proPSA based on varying truncations including [−2] and [−4] proPSA. [−2] proPSA or p2PSA has shown promise as a prostate cancer biomarker as it is not detected in BPH, and in trials increased the AUC from 0.52 for PSA or 0.53 for percentage free PSA to 0.73 [27]. [−2] proPSA has been used preferentially to total or free PSA for prostate cancer detection or biopsy [28–30].

2.1.3. Prostate-specific antigen density (PSAD) test

The PSAD test attempts to add specificity to PSA testing in prostate cancer by determining the amount of PSA produced in relation to size of the gland, as size has been highly correlated with prostate cancer prognosis [31, 32]. Prostate size can be measured with magnetic resonance imaging or transrectal ultrasound by a physician. High density indicates that a small volume prostate is responsible for making a large amount of PSA, and reflective of prostate cancer. In contrast, low density reflects an enlarged prostate, most likely due to BPH that is responsible for the PSA elevation.

2.1.4. PSA velocity

Another factor suggested to provide more accuracy to PSA in ability to predict prostate cancer lies in the rate at which increase is observed, referred to as PSA velocity. PSA testing is performed at routine intervals in men on active surveillance, and elderly men at risk of developing prostate cancer. Elevated PSA is considered in the range of 4.0–10.0 ng/ml, though prostate cancer may still be found in men below this range. PSA velocity factors the rate of PSA increase over time, such that an increase greater than 0.5 ng/ml per year may be indicative of prostate cancer [33].

2.2. The prostate health index

The Prostate Health Index (PHI) is an intuitive formula based upon utilization of several well characterized PSA forms—total PSA, free PSA, and [−2] proPSA or p2PSA, such that:

$$\left(\frac{p2PSA}{free\ PSA}\right) \times \sqrt{PSA} \tag{1}$$

The PHI's multifactorial approach has compounded the precision of each of the PSA measurements providing one patient score, shown to drastically increase the specificity for prostate cancer [28, 34]. PHI has been approved by the FDA for men with PSA in the 4.0–10.0 ng/ml range.

Several clinical trials have retrospectively performed direct comparison to PHI against other early detection biomarkers across blood or urine analysis. In a European cohort of men undergoing either an initial or repeat biopsy, comparing PHI to PSA or free PSA, PHI increased the AUC values to 0.70 compared to 0.65 or 0.53 respectively [35]. In one prospectively performed trial it was determined that 30.1% of patients who underwent a biopsy could have been spared the painful procedure based on PHI score [36]. PHI has additionally been compared against urine biomarkers (to be discussed further in this chapter), with PHI increasing AUC over PCA3 or TMPRSS2:ERG [35, 37]. While results were similar, PHI was the only one correlated with Gleason grade greater than 7 [38].

2.3. The four-Kallikrein panel and 4Kscore® test

The four-kallikrein panel, subsequently referred to as the 4Kscore test is a reflex, or follow-up blood test for men who have an abnormal PSA or digital rectal exam (DRE) result and are being considered for an initial or repeat prostate biopsy after a prior negative biopsy result. True to its name, the test is based upon inclusion of four–kallikreins, total PSA, intact PSA, free PSA in addition to human kallikrein-2 (hK2). The test is generated by OPKO Labs (Nashville, TN) and has been marketed as accurately identifying the risk of aggressive prostate cancer (Gleason >7) in a subsequent biopsy or radical prostatectomy, aiding in patient action plan–based decision making.

The first clinical report of the four-kallikrein panel was among 740 previously unscreened men who underwent biopsy for a PSA above 3.0 ng/ml in the European Randomized Study of Screening for Prostate Cancer [39]. Subsequent studies have been performed for at least 10 cohorts totaling over 15,000 subjects (reviewed in [40]), each of which observed an AUC between 0.80 and 0.90 for the four-kallikrein testing. Results from these studies consistently demonstrate the four-kallikrein panel effectively identified high-grade disease while reducing the number of unnecessary biopsies 49–57% among men being screened for the first time. The 4 k panel is the only test, aside from PSA that has been linked to long-term end-points including prostate cancer metastasis [17, 41]. Studies were initially performed in Europe, and limitations include only retrospective analysis, in primarily white populations with an alternative Gleason scale used. In translation to the United States to incorporate FDA guidelines, modifications of the test were implemented with positive results.

2.4. Stockholm-3

The Stockholm 3 model (S3M) is a combination of blood biomarkers initially including PSA, free PSA, intact PSA, hK2, MSMB, MIC1, genetic polymorphisms (SNPs) and other variabilities such as age, family history, previous prostate biopsies or exam [42, 43]. Later algorithm modification replaced intact PSA with HOXB13 [44]. The goal of the study was to increase the accuracy of high-risk prostate cancer diagnosis. S3M was tested in over 100,000 men, 50–69 years of age with no diagnosis of prostate cancer in Stockholm, Sweden [42, 43]. The performance of S3M was compared to PSA alone. The use of S3M was found to decrease the number of biopsies by more than 50%, avoid negative biopsies and significantly improve the detection of high-risk prostate cancer [42, 43].

2.5. Prostate-specific membrane antigen

Prostate-specific membrane antigen (PSMA) is another glycoprotein with enzymatic function uniquely expressed in the prostate. As its name suggests, what makes it unique from PSA is that it is not a secreted protein, rather it is an integral membrane protein. Yet, like PSA, PSMA is also not specific to prostate cancer.

While PSMA has had little success as a serum based diagnostic marker, it is now being used as the target of an FDA approved radiographic scan (ProstaScint) in which an antibody against PSMA (7E11) is linked to a radiographic agent ^{111}indium. ProstaScint increased predictive value for metastatic prostate cancer, identifying positive lymph node metastases [45]. Several new PSMA specific tracers have been developed for use in PET and PET/CT scanning with performance characteristics that exceed those of ProstaScint and are likely to be approved soon for clinical use.

2.6. Prostatic acid phosphatase

Prostatic acid phosphatase (PAP), or prostatic specific acid phosphatase (PSAP) is a glycoprotein enzyme secreted by prostate cells like PSA. Discovered in the 1930s as a diagnostic biomarker [46], it was replaced with the discovery of PSA in the 1970s. However, PAP reemerged following the discovery that PAP was highly expressed in correlation with tumor staging, and is the target of the first prostate cancer immunotherapy, Sipuleucel-T, approved by the FDA in April, 2010 [47, 48], and which increased overall survival of men with metastatic prostate cancer in its first IMPACT trial [49].

2.7. AR-V7

Androgen receptor splice variant 7 (AR-V7) is a splice variant of androgen receptor (AR) that lacks the ligand binding domain leading to its constitutive transcriptional activity independent of androgens. Due to its androgen independent function, AR-V7 has been implicated in the resistance to second-generation anti-androgen therapies. AR-V7 can be detected in circulating tumor cells (CTCs) and its presence is correlated with resistance to second generation anti-androgens including enzalutamide and abiraterone [50, 51]. These results suggest the use of AR-V7 as a treatment selection biomarker.

3. Tissue-based biomarkers

Tissue based prognosticators are among the most diverse in functionality. Tissue based assays can be performed from as little tissue as a single core of a biopsy up to radical prostatectomy. Yet, these assays are the most invasive due to the nature of tissue extraction through surgical resection or biopsy. Patients may undergo one or multiple sets of biopsies in the course of disease detection and active surveillance. Biomarker screening may also be performed on patients post radical prostatectomy to predict treatment response, recurrence free survival and likelihood of disease progression. Many of these tests are commercial panels available to analyze multiple mRNA signatures in the prostate, but recent advancements in protein and cancer epigenetics are expanding the possibilities of prostate cancer prognosis. Assays are monitored by The National Comprehensive Cancer Network (NCCN), an alliance of U.S. cancer centers directing clinical practice guidelines, as well as the Food and Drug Administration (FDA).

Here we will discuss several of the most commonly used tests:

3.1. DNA

Deoxyribonucleic acid (DNA) is the genetic material of all living things. In comparison to other cancers, prostate cancer has little in the way of genetic mutations. Researchers have used the several well described genomic alterations to their advantage as prognosticators of disease.

3.1.1. Epigenetic testing

Current biopsy strategies sample areas of the prostate in a gridded fashion in attempt to have the most representative assessment of the prostate. Even with this strategy in place, less than 1% of the prostate is sampled. As less than one-third of biopsies return positive results for cancer, there is large concern over inconclusive biopsy results.

The field cancerization effect was first observed in the 1950s when it was noticed that tissues surrounding cancerous lesions contained markers associated with tumor development of oral squamous-cell carcinoma [52]. This phenomenon has since been observed in most solid tumors. Further understanding of the concept is explained in [53]. Today, field effect can translate to modifications in cellular morphology, epigenetics, genomic or mitochondrial DNA alterations, and changes in gene expression or protein levels (reviewed in [54]).

One such assay, ConfirmMDx, tests the epigenetic field effect by observing the molecular changes in methylations occurring in prostate cancer. DNA methylation is among the most common measures of epigenetic abnormality, and easiest to test. These alterations are not detectable in histological analyses, but visible with methylation specific PCR (MSP). Biologically these methylations may be responsible for silencing of key tumor-suppressive genes critical to preventing cancer development, and because of the cancer field effect, this test dramatically amplifies the tested area of the prostate. ConfirmMDx is recommended for men having undergone an initial negative biopsy.

Prostate cancer-associated epigenetic biomarkers used in this assay include glutathione S-transferase-Pi (GSTP1), APC and RASSF1. Methylation of GSTP1 is among the most common somatic alterations observed in prostate cancer with high specificity and sensitivity, and which correlates strongly with Gleason score, age, PSA and DRE [55–57].

3.1.2. PTEN loss and ERG rearrangements

Phosphatase and tensin homolog (PTEN) is a tumor suppressor commonly lost in many cancers. Loss of PTEN is one of few genomic alterations occurring in prostate cancer. PTEN deletion associates with poor outcome and is an established prognostic biomarker for prostate cancer. Analysis of prostatic tissue by Immunohistochemistry (IHC) or Fluorescence in situ hybridization (FISH) demonstrated that PTEN loss is associated with prostate cancer biochemical recurrence, disease progression and metastasis [58–63].

TMPRSS2:ERG fusion is found in ~50% of prostate cancer [64, 65]. TMPRSS2:ERG is a result of gene rearrangement and fusion between androgen regulated transmembrane protease, serine 2 (TMPRSS2) and ERG transcriptional factor genes [64, 65]. This leads to significant overexpression of ERG reported to promote prostate cancer oncogenesis [66–70]. TMPRSS2-ERG rearrangements are accompanied by PTEN loss, which cooperates to promote prostate cancer progression [69, 70]. Moreover, loss of PTEN and presence of TMPRSS2:ERG fusion together predict prostate cancer biochemical recurrence [71] and Metamark further provides screening for loss of PTEN and ERG rearrangement in their PTEN/ERG screen.

3.2. mRNA

Messenger RNA or ribonucleic acid (mRNA) is genetic material carrying information between DNA and protein.

3.2.1. The genomic prostate score

Oncotype DX offers a diverse array of genomic health testing including breast, colon and prostate cancer. The Genomic Prostate Score (GPS) is a prostate specific array which aids in decision-making between initiating immediate treatment or active surveillance. The test measures expression from 12 genes in four prostate cancer associated biological pathways: androgen signaling (AZGP1, FAM13C, KLK2, SRD5A2), cellular organization (FLNC, GSN, GSTM2, TPM2), stromal response (BGN, COL1A1, SFRP4) and cellular proliferation (TPX2), as well as 5 reference genes (ARF1, ATF5E, CLTC, GPS1, PGK1) [72]. This assay has been validated prospectively as an independent predictor of tumor aggressiveness based on adverse pathology, and death associated with prostate cancer and metastasis [73, 74]. GPS is advised for patients with low-risk clinical prostate cancer (very low, low or intermediate NCCN risk). AZGP1 was further validated as a potential biomarker for significant disease [75]. Loss of AZGP1 assessed by RNA in situ hybridization and immunohistochemical analysis is associated with worse outcome and overall survival [75].

3.2.2. Prolaris

Prolaris is a prognostic genetic test developed by Myria Genetic Laboratories based on a 46-gene expression signature strongly tied to cell cycle progression genes. Uniquely paired with cellular proliferation and Gleason grading, The Prolaris Score is generated as a metric of an individual's prostate cancer aggressiveness. This score provides a relative risk among patients of the same risk group defined by the American Urological Association (AUA), and a 10-year prostate cancer specific mortality risk in men with localized disease [76].

3.2.3. Decipher

The Decipher Biopsy was generated from GenomeDX, based on whole genome technology. In men with localized prostate cancer undergoing biopsy or radical prostatectomy, this test divides patients into Low Risk or High Risk, aiding clinicians and patients in decision making toward active surveillance or intensification of treatment with multi-modal therapies. Decipher Biopsy measures 22 RNA biomarkers to correlate the probability of clinical metastasis within 5 years following radical prostatectomy [77] and is predictive of lymph node metastasis [78]. This test can be performed on either biopsy or prostatectomy samples reproducibly [79].

3.3. Protein

3.3.1. ProMark

ProMark is the first protein based prognostic test for prostate cancer from Metamark Genetics Inc. Based on the understanding that mRNA levels may not be completely reflective of a diseased state, ProMark assays protein levels in intact, formalin fixed biopsy samples to infer prognostic information about the patients' condition at the time of biopsy. Based on a quantitative multiplex immunofluorescence (QMPI) platform in which tissues are fixed in formalin, samples are stained for eight protein markers for cancer and normal regions and quantified in situ [80]. Markers include SMAD4, PDSS2, HSPA9, FIS, pS6, and YBOX1 to designate regions of prostate cancer, as well as proteins found in tumor and benign tissues, DERL1 and CUL2. Selected by computational modeling, these combinations of protein markers reflect the morphology from tumor epithelium for reliable prognostication [80–82]. Cost to perform ProMark protein screening is additionally quite low compared to usual guideline-based care [83]. ProMark has been utilized in clinical studies to predict lethal outcome. The test is currently recommended for men with Gleason grade 3 + 3 or 3 + 4 prostate cancer as part of the NCCN Clinical Care Guidelines.

3.3.2. p63 and AMACR

p63 has been identified as a marker of basal cells in multiple epithelial tissues including normal prostate [84]. Significant downregulation or loss p63 is commonly observed in prostate cancer [84, 85]. Alpha-methylacyl coenzyme A racemase (AMACR) is commonly found overexpressed in prostate cancer and exhibits little to no expression in the normal prostate tissues [86–89]. A combination of high-molecular weight cytokeratins, AMACR and loss of p63 can be used to define normal prostate tissues, prostate intraepithelial neoplasia and prostate adenocarcinoma [90, 91].

4. Urine biomarkers

Urine analysis is a non-invasive screening technique for prostate cancer.

4.1. PCA3

Prostate cancer antigen 3 (PCA3) (also known as DD3) is a non-coding mRNA specifically expressed in human prostate tissues, and highly overexpressed in prostate cancer [92].

The Progensa PCA3 assay is an FDA approved urine based molecular test to aid in repeat biopsy decisions from Hologic [93]. Following DRE, a simple "first-catch" urine test captures prostate epithelial cells released into the urine. PCA3 mRNA levels are quantified in proportion to PSA. Also included in the NCCN's Clinical Practice guidelines for prostate cancer early detection, this test's specificity lies in PCA3 which is highly upregulated in prostate cancer cells and not affected by instances of benign prostatic hyperplasia (BPH), prostatitis or other conditions as is the case for PSA. PCA3 testing is currently FDA approved for men previously having a negative biopsy with a persistently elevated PSA to help identify men who need a repeat biopsy. PCA3 is calibrated to identify men at low risk for a positive biopsy such that PCA3 < 25 indicates that it is safe to forgo the biopsy. Increase in score was directly correlated with likelihood of positive repeat biopsies, and predictive of 4-year biopsy outcome [94–96]. PCA3 has subsequently been explored and proven to positively predict detection of prostate cancer in initial biopsies with high specificity and may aid in initial biopsy decision making [97, 98].

4.2. SelectMDX

Utilizing first catch post-DRE urine, SelectMDx tests for mRNA levels of genes DLX1 and HOXC6. Analysis for this test incorporates multifactorial data from PSA density and prior biopsy data to increase significance of this liquid biopsy. This test has shown promise over PCA3 in two prospective clinical trials in identification of patients with high-grade prostate cancer (AUC of 0.90 in first cohort and 0.86 in validation cohort) [99]. SelectMDx was recently added to the European Association of Urology's list for added decision making before a repeat biopsy.

4.3. TMPRSS2:ERG

As ERG rearrangements occur at the genomic level, prostate cancer associated gene fusions such as TMPRSS2:ERG rearrangements are also detectable in patient urine [71, 86–89]. Urine TMPRSS2:ERG was found to associate with Gleason score and tumor size in a large multicenter study with 1312 men [100]. This strategy utilizes transcription mediated amplification (TMA) assay to quantify TMPRSS2-ERG mRNA normalized to PSA mRNA. Additionally, it was demonstrated that the combination of urine TMPRSS2:ERG with urine PCA3, improves the performance of serum PSA for predicting prostate cancer risk [100–102].

4.4. Mi-prostate score (MiPS)

The Michigan Prostate Score (MiPS) combines serum PSA levels with urine analysis for TMPRSS2:ERG and PCA3 mRNA as a predictive model for a positive prostate cancer biopsy. This compounded analysis of three independent prostate markers are closely correlated with presence of prostate cancer in an initial or repeat biopsy and provides a more accurate predictive model of biopsy detected prostate cancer [101].

4.5. Extracellular vesicles

Exosomes are small extracellular vesicles secreted from cells ranging in size from 30 to 120 nm. A portion of the parent cell cytoplasm is contained inside each exosome for the biological function of cell-to-cell communication. For the purpose of clinical diagnostics, this mechanism can be manipulated to measure exosomal genetic material released into blood, urine or other biological fluids. RNA expression from tumor cells is promising as they are highly representative of cell of origin. As exosomes are secreted freely into the urine, exosomal based testing does not require biopsies to detect oncogenic signatures [103, 104]. For instance, PCA3 and ERG mRNAs can be detected in exosomes and be predictive for high grade prostate cancer [105].

4.6. ExoDX prostate (IntelliScore)

Exosomal analysis of PCA3 and ERG RNA copy number from prostate cancer patient urine was determined to positively predict presence of high-grade prostate cancer [105, 106]. This test, now marketed as ExoDX *Prostate(IntelliScore)* is considered a liquid biopsy, combining urine with PSA screening from blood sample. Clinically, *Prostate(IntelliScore)* correctly predicts the occurrence of Gleason scores above 7, and has been recommended for men over 50 with PSA levels in the 2–10 ng/ml range. Further evaluation of this biomarker assay is currently underway.

New technologies are expanding to increase the capture and analysis for extracellular vesicles as experimental material. Exosome Diagnostics, who market the ***Prostate(IntelliScore)*** additionally provide isolation kids for exosomal RNA. Alternatively, devices such as the Exosome Total Isolation Chip (ExoTIC), have been generated specific for the high-yield isolation of extracellular vesicles from biofluids (blood, urine, and lavage), even allowing for separation among vesicles based on size. This work has initially been applied to protein and microRNA analysis, increasing the scope of assayable markers for prostate cancer [107].

5. Conclusions

Assays and technologies have vastly improved prediction strategies for recurrent prostate cancer and metastatic disease. Collectively, the biomarkers and assays presented within this chapter represent great advances in the diagnosis and prognostic assessment of patients with prostate cancer and aid in decision-making for subsequent treatment strategies (reviewed in **Table 1**). However, even with this extensive armamentarium there is still improvement to be made in risk-stratification to accurately identify patients with cancer, and among them, those at risk of developing high grade disease. As biomarkers become available it is increasingly important to understand how these tests are helpful to know when and on which patients these tests should be utilized. Guidelines for care are consistently monitored by urological associations globally. While recommendations vary based on country and among individual institutions and providers, more than ever, patient led decision making is at the forefront of screening. This was evidenced by USPSTF's recent removal of PSA screening for healthy men as routine procedure, instead recommending individualized decision-making by physician counseling of patients as to the potential risks of inaccurate diagnosis leading to over-treatment.

Human nature understandably dictates a need for testing to be as minimally invasive as possible to eliminate painful procedures, and increase patient compliance and willingness to participate in early disease screening. The development of non-invasive screening methods such as blood and urine assays to limit prostate biopsy aids in reducing painful, and in the case of prostate cancer, often unnecessary procedures. This is even further amplified when taken into account the number of men who have to undergo the biopsy procedure repeatedly in the course of diagnosis and disease progression. The future of cancer screening, and hopefully diagnosis will come

Test	Specimen	Invasive	Implication	Biomarkers tested	Genetic Material Tested	FDA Status	Sources
PSA	Blood	Non-invasive	Treatment response and progression free survival	PSA	Protein	Approved	[10-33]
Prostate Health Index (PHI)	Blood	Non-invasive	Risk-assessment and repeat biopsy decision	total PSA, free PSA, [-2]proPSA	Protein	Approved	[28,34-38]
4Kscore	Blood	Non-invasive	Risk-assessment	total PSA, intact PSA, free PSA, hK2	Protein	total PSA, free PSA- Approved; 4kscore- CLIA	[17,39-41]
Stockholm-3	Blood	Non-invasive	Risk-assessment	PSA, free PSA, hK2, MSMB, MIC1, HOXB13, clinical variables, genetic markers and prostate examination	Protein/DNA	None	[42-44]
AR-V7	Blood	Non-invasive	Therapy resistance	AR-V7	RNA	CLIA	[50,51]
ConfirmMDx	Tissue	Invasive	Risk-assessment and repeat biopsy decision	Methylated GSTP1, APC and RASSF1	DNA	CLIA	[55-57]
PTEN/TMPRSS2:ERG	Tissue	Invasive	Risk-assessment and treatment planning	PTEN and ERG	DNA	CLIA	[58-71]
Oncotype DX Genomic Prostate Score	Tissue	Invasive	Risk-assessment and treatment planning	AZGP1, FAM13C, KLK2, SRD5A2, FLNC, GSN, GSTM2, TPM2, BGN, COL1A1, SFRP4, TPX2	RNA	CLIA	[72-75]
Prolaris	Tissue	Invasive	Risk-assessment and treatment planning	46 RNA biomarkers, Gleason score	RNA	CLIA	[76]
Decipher	Tissue	Invasive	Treatment planning	22 RNA biomarkers	RNA	CLIA	[77-79]
ProMark	Tissue	Invasive	Risk-assessment and treatment planning	SMAD4, PDSS2, HSPA9, FUS, pS6, YBOX1, DERL1, CUL2	Protein	CLIA	[80-84]
Progensa	DRE Urine/Blood	Non-invasive	Risk-assessment and repeat biopsy decision	PCA3 and PSA	RNA/Protein	Approved	[92-98]
SelectMDx	DRE Urine/Blood	Non-invasive	Repeat biopsy decision	DLX1, HOXC6 and PSA	RNA/Protein	Exempt	[99]
TMPRSS2:ERG	Urine	Non-invasive	Risk-assessment	TMPRSS2:ERG	RNA	CLIA	[71][86-89][100-102]
MiPS	Urine/Blood	Non-invasive	Risk-assessment	TMPRSS2:ERG, PCA3, PSA	RNA/Protein	CLIA	[101]
ExoDX Prostate (Intelliscore)	Urine/Blood	Non-invasive	Risk-assessment, active surveillance monitoring	ERG, PCA3, PSA	Exosomal RNA	Exempt	[105-107]

Table 1. Screening assays for prostate cancer, classified by specimen and genetic material tested, invasiveness of the assay, clinical uses, biomarkers tested, and status of FDA approval. Certain tests have been proven exempt from FDA regulations, and these are also specified. The Clinical Laboratory Improvement Amendments (CLIA) certifies clinical laboratory developed tests to perform additional testing.

from less invasive procedures. One such advance may be the implementation of imaging strategies such as multi-parametric magnetic resonance imaging (mpMRI) to locate and diagnose prostate cancer. Offered prior to biopsy, patients with negative results are spared the biopsy, while those with cancerous lesions can undergo a targeted biopsy aided by mpMRI, minimizing complications, and obtaining accurate biopsies with ample cancer tissue to aid in treatment plan determination. This technique has tested more accurate than standard of care transrectal ultrasound (TRUS) biopsy in predicting presence of aggressive prostate cancer [108]. The role of imaging in prostate cancer diagnosis is still evolving and these technologies stand to introduce new avenues to the field of prostate cancer diagnosis and even treatment which may lead to better patient risk-stratification with increased survival rates of aggressive prostate cancer.

Acknowledgements

This chapter is written in dedication to Gerald Robert Howley.

The authors thank James D. Brooks for helpful comments and review.

T.S. is supported by the National Institute of Health/National Cancer Institute and Stanford McCormick-Gabilan Faculty Award.

Conflict of interest

The authors declare no conflicts.

Author details

Meghan A. Rice and Tanya Stoyanova*

*Address all correspondence to: stanya@stanford.edu

Department of Radiology, Canary Center for Cancer Early Detection, Stanford University, Palo Alto, CA, USA

References

[1] Siegel RL, Miller KD, Jemal A. Cancer statistics. CA: A Cancer Journal for Clinicians. 2018;**68**(1):7-30

[2] Campos-Fernandes J-L, Bastien L, Nicolaiew N, Robert G, Terry S, Vacherot F, et al. Prostate cancer detection rate in patients with repeated extended 21-sample needle biopsy. European Urology. 2009 Mar;**55**(3):600-606

[3] Nam RK, Saskin R, Lee Y, Liu Y, Law C, Klotz LH, et al. Increasing hospital admission rates for urological complications after transrectal ultrasound guided prostate biopsy. The Journal of Urology. 2013;**189**(1 Suppl):S12-S17; discussion S17-8

[4] Loeb S, Vellekoop A, Ahmed HU, Catto J, Emberton M, Nam R, et al. Systematic review of complications of prostate biopsy. European Urology. 2013;**64**:876-892

[5] Wade J, Rosario DJ, Macefield RC, Avery KNL, Salter CE, Goodwin ML, et al. Psychological impact of prostate biopsy: Physical symptoms, anxiety, and depression. Journal of Clinical Oncology. 2013;**31**(33):4235-4241

[6] Andriole GL, Crawford ED, Grubb RL, Buys SS, Chia D, Church TR, et al. Prostate cancer screening in the randomized prostate, lung, colorectal, and ovarian cancer screening trial: Mortality results after 13 years of follow-up. Journal of the National Cancer Institute. 2012;**104**(2):125-132

[7] Strimbu K, Tavel JA. What are biomarkers? Current Opinion in HIV and AIDS. 2011; **5**(6):463-466

[8] Hanley A, Mcneil J. The meaning and use of the area under a receiver operating characteristic (ROC) curve. Radiology. 1982;**143**:29-36

[9] Albitar M, Ma W, Lund L, Albitar F, Diep K, Fritsche HA, et al. Predicting prostate biopsy results using a panel of plasma and urine biomarkers combined in a scoring system. Journal of Cancer. 2016;**7**(3):297-303

[10] Ablin RJ, Soanes A, Bronson P, Witebsky E. Precipitating antigens of the normal human prostate. Journal of Reproduction and Fertility. 1970;**22**(December 1969):573-574

[11] Lucia MS, Darke AK, Goodman PJ, La Rosa FG, Parnes HL, Ford LG, et al. Pathologic characteristics of cancers detected in the prostate cancer prevention trial: Implications for prostate cancer detection and chemoprevention. Cancer Prevention Research. 2008;**1**:167-173

[12] Thompson IM, Pauler DK, Goodman PJ, Tangen CM, Lucia MS, Parnes HL, et al. Prevalence of prostate cancer among men with a prostate-specific antigen level < or =4.0 ng per milliliter. The New England Journal of Medicine. 2004;**350**(22):2239-2246

[13] Miller DC, Gruber SB, Hollenbeck BK, Montie JE, Wei JT. Incidence of initial local therapy among men with lower-risk prostate cancer in the United States. Journal of the National Cancer Institute. 2006;**98**(16):1134-1141

[14] Moyer VA. Screening for prostate cancer: U.S. preventive services task force recommendation statement. Annals of Internal Medicine. 2012;**157**:120-134

[15] Lilja H, Christensson A, Dahlen U, Matikainen MT, Nilsson O, Pettersson K, et al. Prostate-specific antigen in serum occurs predominantly in complex with α1-antichymotrypsin. Clinical Chemistry. 1991;**37**(9):1618-1625

[16] Rannikko S, Tuhkanen K, Alfthan O. A complex between prostate-specific antigen and α1-antichymotrypsin is the major form of prostate-specific antigen in serum of patients with prostatic cancer: Assay of the complex improves clinical sensitivity for cancer. Cancer Research. 1991;**51**(1):222-226

[17] Steuber T, Nurmikko P, Haese A, Pettersson K, Graefen M, Hammerer P, et al. Discrimination of benign from malignant prostatic disease by selective measurements of single chain, intact free prostate specific antigen. The Journal of Urology. 2002;**168**(5):1917-1922

[18] Finne P, Finne R, Bangma C, Hugosson J, Hakama M, Auvinen A, et al. Algorithms based on prostate-specific antigen (PSA), free PSA, digital rectal examination and prostate

volume reduce false-positive PSA results in prostate cancer screening. International Journal of Cancer. 2004;**111**(2):310-315

[19] Mikolajczyk SD, Rittenhouse HG. Tumor-associated forms of prostate specific antigen improve the discrimination of prostate cancer from benign disease. Rinsho Byori. 2004;**52**(3):223-230

[20] Lilja H. Biology of prostate-specific antigen. Urology. 2003;**62**:27-33

[21] Christensson A, Björk T, Nilsson O, Dahlén U, Matikainen MT, Cockett AT, et al. Serum prostate specific antigen complexed to alpha 1-antichymotrypsin as an indicator of prostate cancer. The Journal of Urology. 1993;**150**(1):100-105

[22] Catalona WJ, Smith DS. Cancer recurrence and survival rates after anatomic radical retropubic prostatectomy for prostate cancer: Intermediate-term results. The Journal of Urology. 1998;**160**(6 Pt 2):2428-2434

[23] Djavan B, Remzi M, Zlotta AR, Ravery V, Hammerer P, Reissigl A, et al. Complexed prostate-specific antigen, complexed prostate-specific antigen density of total and transition zone, complexed/total prostate-specific antigen ratio, free-to-total prostate-specific antigen ratio, density of total and transition zone prostate-sp. Urology. 2002;**60**(4 Suppl 1):4-9

[24] Khan MA, Sokoll LJ, Chan DW, Mangold LA, Mohr P, Mikolajczyk SD, et al. Clinical utility of proPSA and "benign" PSA when percent free PSA is less than 15%. Urology. 2004;**64**(6):1160-1164

[25] Mikolajczyk SD, Grauer LS, Millar LS, Hill TM, Kumar A, Rittenhouse HG, et al. A precursor form of PSA (pPSA) is a component of the free PSA in prostate cancer serum. Urology. 1997;**50**(5):710-714

[26] Mikolajczyk SD, Millar LS, Wang TJ, Rittenhouse HG, Marks LS, Song W, et al. A precursor form of prostate-specific antigen is more highly elevated in prostate cancer compared with benign transition zone prostate tissue. Cancer Research. 2000;**60**(3):756-759

[27] Sokoll LJ, Wang Y, Feng Z, Kagan J, Partin AW, Sanda MG, et al. [−2]proenzyme prostate specific antigen for prostate cancer detection: A national cancer institute early detection research network validation study. The Journal of Urology. 2008;**180**(2):539-543; discussion 543

[28] Loeb S, Catalona WJ. The prostate health index: A new test for the detection of prostate cancer. Therapeutic Advances in Urology. 2014;**6**(2):74-77

[29] Catalona WJ, Bartsch G, Rittenhouse HG, Evans CL, Linton HJ, Amirkhan A, et al. Serum pro prostate specific antigen improves cancer detection compared to free and complexed prostate specific antigen in men with prostate specific antigen 2 to 4 ng/ml. The Journal of Urology. 2003;**170**(6 I):2181-2185

[30] Sokoll LJ, Sanda MG, Feng Z, Kagan J, Mizrahi IA, Broyles DL, et al. A prospective, multicenter, national cancer institute early detection research network study of [−2]proPSA: Improving prostate cancer detection and correlating with cancer aggressiveness. Cancer Epidemiology, Biomarkers & Prevention. 2010;**19**(5):1193-1200

[31] Benson MC, Seong Whang I, Pantuck A, Ring K, Kaplan SA, Olsson CA, et al. Prostate specific antigen density: A means of distinguishing benign prostatic hypertrophy and prostate cancer. The Journal of Urology. 1992;**147**(3):815-816

[32] Benson MC, McMahon DJ, Cooner WH, Olsson CA. An algorithm for prostate cancer detection in a patient population using prostate-specific antigen and prostate-specific antigen density. World Journal of Urology. 1993;**11**(4):206-213

[33] Vickers AJ, Brewster SF. PSA velocity and doubling time in diagnosis and prognosis of prostate cancer. British Journal of Medical and Surgical Urology. 2012;**5**:162-168

[34] Catalona WJ, Partin AW, Sanda MG, Wei JT, Klee GG, Bangma CH, et al. A multicenter study of [−2]pro-prostate specific antigen combined with prostate specific antigen and free prostate specific antigen for prostate cancer detection in the 2.0 to 10.0 ng/ml prostate specific antigen range. The Journal of Urology. 2011;**185**(5):1650-1655

[35] Scattoni V, Lazzeri M, Lughezzani G, De Luca S, Passera R, Bollito E, et al. Head-to-head comparison of prostate health index and urinary PCA3 for predicting cancer at initial or repeat biopsy. The Journal of Urology. 2013 Aug 1;**190**(2):496-501

[36] Loeb S, Sanda MG, Broyles DL, Shin SS, Bangma CH, Wei JT, et al. The prostate health index selectively identifies clinically significant prostate cancer. The Journal of Urology. 2015;**193**(4):1163-1169

[37] Ferro M, Bruzzese D, Perdonà S, Marino A, Mazzarella C, Perruolo G, et al. Prostate health index (phi) and prostate cancer antigen 3 (PCA3) significantly improve prostate cancer detection at initial biopsy in a total PSA range of 2-10 ng/ml. PLoS One. 2013;**8**(7):1-7

[38] Stephan C, Vincendeau S, Houlgatte A, Cammann H, Jung K, Semjonow A. Multicenter evaluation of [−2]proprostate-specific antigen and the prostate health index for detecting prostate cancer. Clinical Chemistry [Internet]. 2013 Jan 1;**59**(1):306-314. Available from: http://clinchem.aaccjnls.org/content/59/1/306.abstract

[39] Vickers AJ, Till C, Tangen CM, Lilja H, Thompson IM. An empirical evaluation of guidelines on prostate-specific antigen velocity in prostate cancer detection. Journal of the National Cancer Institute. 2011;**103**(6):462-469

[40] Punnen S, Pavan N, Parekh DJ. Finding the wolf in sheep's clothing: The 4Kscore is a novel blood test that can accurately identify the risk of aggressive prostate cancer. Revista de Urología. 2015;**17**(1):3-13

[41] Stattin P, Vickers AJ, Sjoberg DD, Johansson R, Granfors T, Johansson M, et al. Improving the specificity of screening for lethal prostate cancer using prostate-specific antigen and a panel of Kallikrein markers: A nested case–control study. European Urology. 2015 Aug;**68**(2):207-213

[42] Eklund M, Nordström T, Aly M, Adolfsson J, Wiklund P, Brandberg Y, et al. The Stockholm-3 (STHLM3) model can improve prostate cancer diagnostics in men aged 50-69 yr compared with current prostate cancer testing. European Urology Focus. 2016;**229**:1-4

[43] Grönberg H, Adolfsson J, Aly M, Nordström T, Wiklund P, Brandberg Y, et al. Prostate cancer screening in men aged 50-69 years (STHLM3): A prospective population-based diagnostic study. The Lancet Oncology. 2015;**16**(16):1667-1676

[44] Ström P, Nordström T, Grönberg H, Eklund M. The Stockholm-3 model for prostate cancer detection: Algorithm update, biomarker contribution, and reflex test potential. European Urology. 2018;**7687**:1-7

[45] Rieter WJ, Keane TE, Ahlman MA, Ellis CT, Spicer KM, Gordon LL. Diagnostic performance of In-111 capromab pendetide SPECT/CT in localized and metastatic prostate cancer. Clinical Nuclear Medicine. 2011;**36**(10):872-878

[46] Gutman AB, Gutman EB. An "acid" phosphatase occurring in the serum of patients with metastasizing carcinoma of the prostate gland. The Journal of Clinical Investigation. 1938;**17**(4):473-478

[47] Huber ML, Haynes L, Parker C, Iversen P. Interdisciplinary critique of Sipuleucel-T as immunotherapy in castration-resistant prostate cancer. Journal of the National Cancer Institute. 2012;**104**:273-279

[48] Gerritsen WR. The evolving role of immunotherapy in prostate cancer. Annals of Oncology. 2012;**23**(Suppl 8):viii22-vvii27

[49] Kantoff PW, Higano CS, Shore ND, Berger ER, Small EJ, Penson DF, et al. Sipuleucel-T immunotherapy for castration-resistant prostate cancer. The New England Journal of Medicine. 2010;**363**(5):411-422

[50] Antonarakis ES, Lu C, Wang H, Luber B, Nakazawa M, Roeser JC, et al. AR-V7 and resistance to enzalutamide and abiraterone in prostate cancer. The New England Journal of Medicine. 2014;**371**(11):1028-1038

[51] Antonarakis ES, Lu C, Luber B, Wang H, Chen Y, Zhu Y, et al. Clinical significance of androgen receptor splice variant-7 mRNA detection in circulating tumor cells of men with metastatic castration-resistant prostate cancer treated with first- and second-line abiraterone and enzalutamide. Journal of Clinical Oncology. 2017;**35**(19):2149-2156

[52] Slaughter DP, Southwick HW, Smejkal W. "Field cancerization" in oral stratified squamous epithelium. Clinical implications of multicentric origin. Cancer. 1953;**6**(5):963-968

[53] Braakhuis BJM, Tabor MP, Kummer JA, Leemans CR, Brakenhoff RH. A genetic explanation of slaughter's concept of field cancerization. Cancer Research. 2003;**63**(8):1727-1730

[54] Trujillo KA, Jones AC, Griffith JK, Bisoffi M. Markers of field cancerization: Proposed clinical applications in prostate biopsies. Prostate Cancer. 2012 May 14;**2012**:302894

[55] Lee WH, Morton RA, Epstein JI, Brooks JD, Campbell PA, Bova GS, et al. Cytidine methylation of regulatory sequences near the pi-class glutathione S-transferase gene accompanies human prostatic carcinogenesis. Proceedings of the National Academy of Sciences. 1994;**91**(24):11733-11737

[56] Zhou M, Tokumaru Y, Sidransky D, Epstein JI. Quantitative GSTP1 methylation levels correlate with Gleason grade and tumor volume in prostate needle biopsies. The Journal of Urology. 2004;**171**(6, Part 1):2195-2198

[57] Van Neste L, Herman JG, Otto G, Bigley JW, Epstein JI, Van Criekinge W. The epigenetic promise for prostate cancer diagnosis. The Prostate. 2012;**72**:1248-1261

[58] Lotan TL, Wei W, Ludkovski O, Morais CL, Guedes LB, Jamaspishvili T, et al. Analytic validation of a clinical-grade PTEN immunohistochemistry assay in prostate cancer by comparison with PTEN FISH. Modern Pathology. 2016;**29**(8):904-914

[59] Lotan TL, Heumann A, Dwertmann Rico S, Hicks J, Lecksell K, Koop C, et al. PTEN loss detection in prostate cancer: Comparison of PTEN immunohistochemistry and PTEN FISH in a large retrospective prostatectomy cohort. Oncotarget. 2017;**2**(2):180-188

[60] Lotan TL, Wei W, Morais CL, Hawley ST, Fazli L, Hurtado-Coll A, et al. PTEN loss as determined by clinical-grade immunohistochemistry assay is associated with worse recurrence-free survival in prostate cancer. European Urology Focus. 2016;**2**(2):180-188

[61] Lotan TL, Carvalho FL, Peskoe SB, Hicks JL, Good J, Fedor HL, et al. PTEN loss is associated with upgrading of prostate cancer from biopsy to radical prostatectomy. Modern Pathology. 2015;**28**(1):128-137

[62] Lotan TL, Gurel B, Sutcliffe S, Esopi D, Liu W, Xu J, et al. PTEN protein loss by immunostaining: Analytic validation and prognostic indicator for a high risk surgical cohort of prostate cancer patients. Clinical Cancer Research. 2011;**17**(20):6563-6573

[63] Chaux A, Peskoe SB, Gonzalez-Roibon N, Schultz L, Albadine R, Hicks J, et al. Loss of PTEN expression is associated with increased risk of recurrence after prostatectomy for clinically localized prostate cancer. Modern Pathology. 2012;**25**(11):1-7

[64] Tomlins SA, Rhodes DR, Perner S, Dhanasekaran SM, Mehra R, Sun X-W, et al. Recurrent fusion of TMPRSS2 and ETS transcription factor genes in prostate cancer. Science. 2005;**310**(5748):644-648

[65] Cancer Genome Atlas Research Network. The molecular taxonomy of primary prostate Cancer. Cell. 2015;**163**(4):1011-1025

[66] Tomlins SA, Bjartell A, Chinnaiyan AM, Jenster G, Nam RK, Rubin MA, et al. ETS gene fusions in prostate cancer: From discovery to daily clinical practice. European Urology. 2009;**56**:275-286

[67] Zong Y, Xin L, Goldstein AS, Lawson DA, Teitell MA, Witte ON. ETS family transcription factors collaborate with alternative signaling pathways to induce carcinoma from adult murine prostate cells. Proceedings of the National Academy of Sciences. 2009;**106**(30):12465-12470

[68] Rostad K, Hellwinkel OJC, Haukaas SA, Halvorsen OJ, Øyan AM, Haese A, et al. TMPRSS2:ERG fusion transcripts in urine from prostate cancer patients correlate with a less favorable prognosis. APMIS. 2009;**117**(8):575-582

[69] King JC, Xu J, Wongvipat J, Hieronymus H, Carver BS, Leung DH, et al. Cooperativity of TMPRSS2-ERG with PI3-kinase pathway activation in prostate oncogenesis. Nature Genetics. 2009;**41**(5):524-526

[70] Carver BS, Tran J, Gopalan A, Chen Z, Shaikh S, Carracedo A, et al. Aberrant ERG expression cooperates with loss of PTEN to promote cancer progression in the prostate. Nature Genetics. 2009;**41**(5):619-624

[71] Yoshimoto M, Joshua AM, Cunha IW, Coudry RA, Fonseca FP, Ludkovski O, et al. Absence of TMPRSS2:ERG fusions and PTEN losses in prostate cancer is associated with a favorable outcome. Modern Pathology. 2008;**21**(12):1451-1460

[72] Klein EA, Cooperberg MR, Magi-Galluzzi C, Simko JP, Falzarano SM, Maddala T, et al. A 17-gene assay to predict prostate cancer aggressiveness in the context of Gleason grade heterogeneity, tumor multifocality, and biopsy undersampling. European Urology. 2014;**66**(3):550-560

[73] Cullen J, Rosner IL, Brand TC, Zhang N, Tsiatis AC, Moncur J, et al. A biopsy-based 17-gene genomic prostate score predicts recurrence after radical prostatectomy and adverse surgical pathology in a racially diverse population of men with clinically low- and intermediate-risk prostate cancer. European Urology. 2015;**68**(1):123-131

[74] Knezevic D, Goddard AD, Natraj N, Cherbavaz DB, Clark-Langone KM, Snable J, et al. Analytical validation of the oncotype DX prostate cancer assay—A clinical RT-PCR assay optimized for prostate needle biopsies. BMC Genomics. 2013;**14**(1):1-12

[75] Brooks JD, Wei W, Pollack JR, West RB, Shin JH, Sunwoo JB, et al. Loss of expression of AZGP1 is associated with worse clinical outcomes in a multi-institutional radical prostatectomy cohort. The Prostate. 2016;**76**(15):1409-1419

[76] Cuzick J, Stone S, Fisher G, Yang ZH, North BV, Berney DM, et al. Validation of an RNA cell cycle progression score for predicting death from prostate cancer in a conservatively managed needle biopsy cohort. British Journal of Cancer. 2015;**113**(3):382-389

[77] Klein EA, Haddad Z, Yousefi K, Lam LLC, Wang Q, Choeurng V, et al. Decipher genomic classifier measured on prostate biopsy predicts metastasis risk. Urology. 2016;**90**:148-152

[78] Lee HJ, Yousefi K, Haddad Z, Abdollah F, Lam LLC, Shin H, et al. Evaluation of a genomic classifier in radical prostatectomy patients with lymph node metastasis. Research and Reports in Urology. 2016;**8**:77-84

[79] Knudsen BS, Kim HL, Erho N, Shin H, Alshalalfa M, Lam LLC, et al. Application of a clinical whole-transcriptome assay for staging and prognosis of prostate cancer diagnosed in needle core biopsy specimens. The Journal of Molecular Diagnostics. 2016;**18**(3):395-406

[80] Blume-Jensen P, Berman DM, Rimm DL, Shipitsin M, Putzi M, Nifong TP, et al. Biology of human tumors development and clinical validation of an in situ biopsy-based multimarker assay for risk stratification in prostate cancer. Clinical Cancer Research. 2015;**21**(11):2591-2600

[81] Shipitsin M, Small C, Choudhury S, Giladi E, Friedlander S, Nardone J, et al. Identification of proteomic biomarkers predicting prostate cancer aggressiveness and lethality despite biopsy-sampling error. British Journal of Cancer. 2014;**111**(6):1201-1212

[82] Shipitsin M, Small C, Giladi E, Siddiqui S, Choudhury S, Hussain S, et al. Automated quantitative multiplex immunofluorescence in situ imaging identifies phospho-S6 and phospho-PRAS40 as predictive protein biomarkers for prostate cancer lethality. Proteome Science. 2014;**12**(1):1-13

[83] Roth JA, Ramsey SD, Carlson JJ. Cost-effectiveness of a biopsy-based 8-protein prostate cancer prognostic assay to optimize treatment decision making in Gleason 3 + 3 and 3 + 4 early stage prostate cancer. The Oncologist. 2015;**20**(12):1355-1364

[84] Signoretti S, Waltregny D, Dilks J, Isaac B, Lin D, Garraway L, et al. p63 is a prostate basal cell marker and is required for prostate development. The American Journal of Pathology. 2000;**157**(6):1769-1775

[85] Dhillon PK, Barry M, Stampfer MJ, Perner S, Fiorentino M, Fornari A, et al. Aberrant cytoplasmic expression of p63 and prostate cancer mortality. Cancer Epidemiology, Biomarkers & Prevention. 2009;**18**(2):595-600

[86] Rubin MA, Zhou M, Dhanasekaran SM, Varambally S, Barrette TR, Sanda MG, et al. α-Methylacyl coenzyme a racemase as a tissue biomarker for prostate cancer. Journal of the American Medical Association. 2002;**287**(13):1662

[87] Luo J, Zha S, Gage WR, T a D, Hicks JL, Bennett CJ, et al. Alpha-methylacyl-CoA racemase: A new molecular marker for prostate cancer. Cancer Research. 2002;**62**:2220-2226

[88] Zhou M, Chinnaiyan AM, Kleer CG, Lucas PC, Rubin MA. Alpha-methylacyl-CoA racemase: A novel tumor marker over-expressed in several human cancers and their precursor lesions. The American Journal of Surgical Pathology. 2002;**26**(7):926-931

[89] Wu CL, Yang XJ, Tretiakova M, Patton KT, Halpern EF, Woda BA, et al. Analysis of α-methylacyl-CoA racemase (P504S) expression in high-grade prostatic intraepithelial neoplasia. Human Pathology. 2004;**35**(8):1008-1013

[90] Shah RB, Kunju LP, Shen R, LeBlanc M, Zhou M, Rubin MA. Usefulness of basal cell cocktail (34βE12 + p63) in the diagnosis of atypical prostate glandular proliferations. American Journal of Clinical Pathology. 2004;**122**(4):517-523

[91] Sung M-T, Jiang Z, Montironi R, MacLennan GT, Mazzucchelli R, Cheng L. Alpha-methylacyl-CoA racemase (P504S)/34betaE12/p63 triple cocktail stain in prostatic adenocarcinoma after hormonal therapy. Human Pathology. 2007;**38**(2):332-341

[92] Bussemakers MJG, Van Bokhoven A, Verhaegh GW, Smit FP, Karthaus HFM, Schalken JA, et al. DD3: A new prostate-specific gene, highly overexpressed in prostate cancer. Cancer Research. 1999;**59**(23):5975-5979

[93] Gittelman MC, Hertzman B, Bailen J, Williams T, Koziol I, Henderson RJ, et al. PCA3 molecular urine test as a predictor of repeat prostate biopsy outcome in men with previous negative biopsies: A prospective multicenter clinical study. The Journal of Urology. 2013;**190**(1):64-69

[94] Aubin SMJ, Reid J, Sarno MJ, Blase A, Aussie J, Rittenhouse H, et al. PCA3 molecular urine test for predicting repeat prostate biopsy outcome in populations at risk: Validation in the placebo arm of the Dutasteride REDUCE trial. The Journal of Urology. 2018 Apr 15;**184**(5):1947-1952

[95] Marks LS, Fradet Y, Lim Deras I, Blase A, Mathis J, Aubin SMJ, et al. PCA3 molecular urine assay for prostate cancer in men undergoing repeat biopsy. Urology. 2007;**69**(3):532-535

[96] Haese A, de la Taille A, van Poppel H, Marberger M, Stenzl A, Mulders PFA, et al. Clinical utility of the PCA3 urine assay in European men scheduled for repeat biopsy. European Urology. 2008;**54**(5):1081-1088

[97] De La Taille A, Irani J, Graefen M, Chun F, De Reijke T, Kil P, et al. Clinical evaluation of the PCA3 assay in guiding initial biopsy decisions. The Journal of Urology. 2011;**185**(6):2119-2125

[98] Chevli KK, Duff M, Walter P, Yu C, Capuder B, Elshafei A, et al. Urinary PCA3 as a predictor of prostate cancer in a cohort of 3,073 men undergoing initial prostate biopsy. The Journal of Urology. 2014;**191**(6):1743-1748

[99] Van Neste L, Hendriks RJ, Dijkstra S, Trooskens G, Cornel EB, Jannink SA, et al. Detection of high-grade prostate cancer using a urinary molecular biomarker–based risk score. European Urology. 2016;**70**(5):740-748

[100] Tomlins SA, Aubin SMJ, Siddiqui J, Lonigro RJ, Sefton-Miller L, Miick S, et al. Urine TMPRSS2:ERG fusion transcript stratifies prostate cancer risk in men with elevated serum PSA. Science Translational Medicine. 2011;**3**(94):1-24

[101] Tomlins SA, Day JR, Lonigro RJ, Hovelson DH, Siddiqui J, Kunju LP, et al. Urine TMPRSS2:ERG plus PCA3 for individualized prostate cancer risk assessment. European Urology. 2016;**70**(1):45-53

[102] Leyten GHJM, Hessels D, Jannink SA, Smit FP, de Jong H, Cornel EB, et al. Prospective multicentre evaluation of PCA3 and TMPRSS2-ERG gene fusions as diagnostic and prognostic urinary biomarkers for prostate cancer. European Urology. 2014;**65**(3):534-542

[103] Mitchell PJ, Welton J, Staffurth J, Court J, Mason MD, Tabi Z, et al. Can urinary exosomes act as treatment response markers in prostate cancer? Journal of Translational Medicine. 2009;**7**:1-13

[104] Nilsson J, Skog J, Nordstrand A, Baranov V, Mincheva-Nilsson L, Breakefield XO, et al. Prostate cancer-derived urine exosomes: A novel approach to biomarkers for prostate cancer. British Journal of Cancer. 2009;**100**(10):1603-1607

[105] Donovan MJ, Noerholm M, Bentink S, Belzer S, Skog J, O'Neill V, et al. A molecular signature of PCA3 and ERG exosomal RNA from non-DRE urine is predictive of initial prostate biopsy result. Prostate Cancer and Prostatic Diseases. 2015;**18**(4):370-375

[106] McKiernan J, Donovan MJ, O'Neill V, Bentink S, Noerholm M, Belzer S, et al. A novel urine exosome gene expression assay to predict high-grade prostate cancer at initial biopsy. JAMA Oncology. 2016;**2**(7):882-889

[107] Liu F, Vermesh O, Mani V, Ge TJ, Madsen SJ, Sabour A, et al. The exosome total isolation chip. ACS Nano. 2017;**11**(11):10712-10723

[108] Ahmed HU, El-Shater Bosaily A, Brown LC, Gabe R, Kaplan R, Parmar MK, et al. Diagnostic accuracy of multi-parametric MRI and TRUS biopsy in prostate cancer (PROMIS): A paired validating confirmatory study. Lancet. 2017;**389**(10071):815-822

Section 3

Prostate Diagnosis - PET Imaging

Chapter 3

Pre-Therapeutic Dosimetry Employing Scandium-44 for Radiolabeling PSMA-617

Elisabeth Eppard

Additional information is available at the end of the chapter

http://dx.doi.org/10.5772/intechopen.79157

Abstract

In recent years, the positron emitter scandium-44 moved into the focus of research providing favorable nuclide properties for an application in nuclear medicine. Radiolabeling of PSMA-617 with scandium-44 as diagnostic match for [^{177}Lu]Lu-PSMA-617 instead of gallium-68 would enable pre-therapeutic dosimetry in clinical setting. Due to the chemical similarities of scandium and lutetium, the in vitro and in vivo characteristics of [^{177}Lu]Lu-PSMA-617 are more similar to [^{44}Sc]Sc-PSMA-617 than to the ^{68}Ga-compounds [^{68}Ga]Ga-PSMA-617 or [^{68}Ga]Ga-PSMA-11. [^{44}Sc]Sc-PSMA-617 showed its potential in a clinical setting as a PET imaging agent of prostate cancer providing several advantages over gallium-68 labeled tracers. The longer half-life of the nuclide would allow, for example, an optimized patient management and treatment, long-term or late time point imaging as well as transportation to more distant PET centers. However, especially clinical applications like individual dosimetry or intraoperative applications are still under investigation.

Keywords: scandium-44, PSMA-617, dosimetry, theranostic, castrate-resistant prostate cancer

1. Introduction

Prostate carcinoma is the fourth most common cancer in both sexes combined, the second most common cancer in men, and with an estimated 307,000 deaths in 2012, it is the fifth leading cause of death from cancer in men [1]. While prognosis of prostate carcinoma is good at an early stage, the 5-year survival of patients in advanced stages decreases to 31% [2, 3]. Consequently, a number of studies were conducted developing new strategies against the disease.

As the prostate-specific membrane antigen (PSMA) is overexpressed on prostate carcinoma and the neovasculature of most of the solid tumors but not of normal tissue, it is an attractive target for imaging and therapy [4]. Consequently, the development and the evaluation of small ligands targeting PSMA are the objectives of various studies.

With the introduction of PSMA-617, a further development of PSMA-11, a highly potent theranostic agent found its way into clinical routine where it is used as [^{68}Ga]Ga-PSMA-617 for PET and as [^{177}Lu]Lu-PSMA-617 for therapy of metastatic castrate-resistant prostate cancer (mCRPC). In the last few years, several studies proved the therapeutic efficacy of [^{177}Lu]Lu-PSMA-617 in mCRPC patients [2, 3, 5]. Although [^{177}Lu]Lu-PSMA-617 exhibited a favorable safety profile in mCRPC patients [2, 3, 5–9], adverse effects were due to physiologic expression of PSMA in small intestine, proximal renal tubules and salivary glands are observable [2, 10, 11]. Correspondingly, organs at risk are kidneys as well as salivary and lacrimal glands. First experiences showed that pre-therapeutic dosimetry might support pre-selection of patients as well as improvement of individualized therapy planning [7, 9, 12–15]. In this context, pre-therapeutic estimation of dose delivered to PSMA expressing tissue as well as whole body would be useful to predict therapeutic effect of a certain administered therapeutic activity and facilitate individual dose adjustment [16]. For this purpose, [^{177}Lu]Lu-PSMA-617 planar ± SPECT imaging, employing small amounts of tracer, or [^{68}Ga]Ga-PSMA-617 PET were considered [10–14, 17–19] but both tracers have disadvantages and limitations for dosimetry in a clinical setting.

Current studies on radiolabeling PSMA-617 with the positron emitter scandium-44 demonstrated its similar in vitro and in vivo properties compared with [^{177}Lu]Lu-PSMA-617 [20, 21]. As it is combining the similar pharmacokinetics to [^{177}Lu]Lu-PSMA-617 with more appropriate nuclide characteristics than [^{68}Ga]Ga-PSMA-617, it is assumed to improve pre-therapeutic dosimetry [20, 21].

2. Part I: Radiochemistry

Currently, [^{68}Ga]Ga-PSMA-11 is the most frequently used PET tracer, targeting the prostate-specific membrane antigen, worldwide [22, 23]. Gallium-68 has for PET imaging appropriate decay properties; nevertheless, its disadvantages limit its application.

Its high positron energy compared to fluorine-18 (cf. **Table 1**) leads to images tending to be noisier while its short physical half-life only covers imaging periods of a few hours. Moreover, the differences in coordination chemistry between gallium-68 and lutetium-177 lead to deviations in pharmacokinetics [20]. As a consequence, gallium-68 is not the nuclide of choice for late time imaging, extended dosimetric evaluations as well as intraoperative applications several hours post-injection (p.i.).

From this point of view, scandium-44 is a genuine alternative to gallium-68 and is in the focus of current research [20, 25–30].

Scandium-44 (β^+ = 94%, $\tilde{E}_\beta$ = 0.632 MeV) has a physical half-life of 3.97 h and can be produced on two different ways, via ^{44}Ti/^{44}Sc-generator or cyclotron [30–36]. Another potential advantage of scandium(III) in nuclear medicine is its radioisotope scandium-47 (β^-, primary ⊚-ray of

Positron emitter	Half-life	$\tilde{E}_\beta$	$E_{\beta, max}$
		(MeV)	
^{68}Ga	67.71 min	0.829	1.899
^{44}Sc	3.97 h	0.632	1.474
^{15}O	2.04 min	0.735	1.732
^{18}F	109.77 min	0.250	0.634

Table 1. Comparison of mean ($\tilde{E}_\beta$) and maximum ($E_{\beta, max}$) positron energies of scandium-44 with gallium-68, fluorine-18 and oxygen-15 [24].

159 keV and t½ = 3.3 d) which is suitable for therapeutical application. Constituting a matched pair of radioisotopes real Sc-labeled theranostic radiopharmaceuticals are applicable [28, 31, 37–40].

Scandium-44 can be quantitatively detected via its 511 keV emission. High radioactivities of scandium-44 can be measured in a dose calibrator applying the ^{18}F-setting. But due to different radionuclide characteristics, a multiplication factor has to be used, which is depending on the dose calibrator.

Since the 1980s, several radiolabeling studies with scandium radionuclides have been published [20, 21, 25, 28, 38, 41–44]. Chemically, scandium is similar to Y^{3+} and lanthanides. However, the ionic radius of Sc^{3+} is smaller than that of lanthanides for the coordination number 6 while at the same time, it is larger than any trivalent 3d transition metal cation. The most common coordination number of Sc^{3+} is six; nevertheless, examples for coordination numbers between three and nine exist [45, 46].

In vivo stability of a radiopharmaceutical is a crucial factor for clinical application; macrocyclic ligands are the ligands of choice forming thermodynamically and kinetically stable complexes with trivalent hard metal cations. Chemical and, at the end, biological behavior of the complex and consequently of the radiopharmaceutical depend on structural factors, for example, rigidity, cavity size and nature and number of the donor atoms chelating the metal cation [47]. Due to the similarity between Sc^{3+} and Ga^{3+}, Y^{3+} or trivalent lanthanides, DOTA, a common ligand in nuclear medicine, was evaluated with regard of its usability [48]. The study revealed that the stability constant of [Sc-DOTA] is comparable with those for Y^{3+} or the heaviest lanthanides and higher than those for In^{3+} and Ga^{3+} as well as the eight-coordination geometry of the complex in solution [48].

Together with its four times longer half-life than gallium-68 and its coordination chemistry similar to lutetium-177, scandium-44 enables longer imaging periods covering up to 24 h post injection as well as improved pre-therapeutic dosimetry.

2.1. Production of scandium-44

Scandium-44 can be produced via $^{44}Ti/^{44}Sc$-generator [30, 31, 40]. Despite the advantages of the radionuclide generator system prevents the availability of titanium-44 the production of this generator. Titanium-44 with its half-life of 60 years is only producible with limited yields and at high costs by a small number of facilities [49]. Accordingly, accessibility of the daughter scandium-44 by cyclotron production is an alternative as it provides scandium-44 in sufficiently high yields with radionuclidic purities >99% avoiding the problem of ^{44}Ti-waste management.

2.1.1. Cyclotron production

Growing interest in scandium-44 as alternative to gallium-68 predicated research for production routes providing scandium-44 in the GBq range. Recent intermediate cyclotrons allow an economic production of the radionuclide utilizing p, d or α-particle-induced reactions (cf. **Table 2**) [26, 27, 33, 50–57]. The isomer scandium-44m ($T_{1/2}$ = 58 h) has also nuclide characteristics, which can be useful in nuclear medicine [26, 43].

Recently, the accessibility of scandium-44 via proton irradiation of natural calcium targets was described [53] as well as the employment of enriched calcium targets optimizing radionuclidic purity of the radionuclide produced [52].

Similar experiments performed by bombarding natural calcium targets with protons were reported [53, 55], yielding more than 650 MBq scandium-44 with 95.8% radionuclidic purity [53]. As this method leads to co-production of long-living radionuclidic impurities accounting for unnecessary doses for the patient its usability is limited. To obtain scandium-44 of higher radionuclidic purity enriched [^{44}Ca]$CaCO_3$ target material was found to be optimal [59]. This study also confirmed an optimal ratio of scandium-44m to scandium-44 by irradiating the targets with 9 MeV protons and the possibility to achieve yields in the GBq range utilizing this method [59]. Further refinement leads to reproducible production of GBq-activities of scandium-44 at a cyclotron in excellent quality [56]. As a result of all these investigations towards scandium-44 production, the basis for the introduction of scandium-44 into clinical routine for PET imaging may have been created.

Nuclide production via cyclotron is in need for an efficient separation strategy of the produced radionuclide from the target material. This is necessary to remove bulk metal, which disturbs eventual radiolabeling of PET tracers, to reduce the volume and to recover target material. For this purpose, different methods such as filtration [53] or ion exchange employing chelating resins were investigated [26, 55, 56, 59].

	Reaction	Q (MeV)	E_{th} (MeV)
p	^{44}Ca(p,n)^{44}Sc	−4.43	4.53
d	^{44}Ca(d,2n)^{44}Sc	−6.65	6.96
	^{44}Ca(d,n)^{44}Sc	0.0	0.0
α	^{44}Ca(α,3np)^{44}Sc	−32.73	35.71
	^{43}Ca(α,2np)^{44}Sc	−21.59	23.61
	^{42}Ca(α,np)^{44}Sc	−13.67	14.97

Table 2. Nuclear reaction data for the formation of scandium-44 [58].

2.1.2. The ^{44}Ti/^{44}Sc-generator

Radionuclide generators are an alternative production route to reactors and cyclotron. They exploit radiochemical equilibria (transient or secular) between mother and daughter isotope. This means that the mother isotope has a half-life much greater than or approximately equal to 10 times longer than the half-life of the daughter usable for imaging. As mother and daughter are isotopes of different elements, they are present in different chemical forms and can be relatively easily separated chemically.

Beside the ^{99}Mo/^{99m}Tc-generator, which is still the working horse in nuclear medicine, the relevance of the ^{68}Ge/^{68}Ga-generator continues to increase with recent developments of new potent ^{68}Ga-radiopharmaceuticals for PET imaging. Apart from the cyclotron, scandium-44 can also be produced via ^{44}Ti/^{44}Sc-generator system. Just like the ^{68}Ge/^{68}Ga-generator, there is a secular equilibrium between the long-living mother and the short-living daughter nuclide. Titanium-44 decays via electron capture ($t_{1/2}$ = 59 ± 2 a) [60] into the ground state of scandium-44 which transforms to the stable calcium isotope calcium-44 emitting a positron.

First studies on the design of a ^{44}Ti/^{44}Sc-generator were conducted in the 1960ies and 70ies excluding pharmaceutical aspects [32, 35, 61, 62]. A first 185 MBq ^{44}Ti/^{44}Sc-generator designed for radiopharmaceutical use was described in the last decade [31] as well as a suitable post-processing [40]. An initial preclinical proof of concept study could show that scandium-44 is able to radiolabel a clinical relevant precursor (DOTA-TOC) leading to a stable radiopharmaceutical in good yields as well as the suitability of the generator and post-processing for this purpose [38]. Furthermore, a first clinical application of [^{44}Sc]Sc-DOTA-TOC, radiolabeled with generator-derived scandium-44, was conducted to proof the high potential of the radionuclide for PET imaging [30].

First challenge in the development of the ^{44}Ti/^{44}Sc-generator is the high-yield production of titantium-44 via accelerated particles. Up to now, all attempts building a ^{44}Ti/^{44}Sc-generator described in the literature use the ^{45}Sc(p,2n)^{44}Ti-process, although cyclotrons of high positron flux are necessary, to obtain titanium-44 in relatively low radioactivity yields [31, 32, 35, 61–63]. Before titanium-44 can be used separation from the target material and subsequent purification from residual metallic contaminants is mandatory.

Generally, for the design of a radionuclide generator, several critical radiochemical parameters have to be considered, such as separation strategy, stability of the generator and type of eluate. In context with the ^{44}Ti/^{44}Sc-generator, this means a separation strategy is needed which provides high ^{44}Sc-elution yields combined with low ^{44}Ti-breakthrough employing an eluate which is suitable for subsequent radiolabeling in terms of pH, volume and purity. Additionally, this separation strategy should guarantee high long-term stability of the generator. This is of particular importance for the ^{44}Ti/^{44}Sc-generator compared for example to the ^{99}Mo/^{99m}Tc- or ^{68}Ge/^{68}Ga-generators as usage for many years due to the long physical half-life of titanium-44 is possible.

The ^{44}Ti/^{44}Sc-generator system developed by Filosofov et al. uses the properties of Sc^{III} in oxalic as well as hydrochloric acid as basis of an anion-exchange separation strategy [31]. This concept leads to ^{44}Sc elution yields of 180 MBq in 20 ml 0.005 M $H_2C_2O_4$/0.07 M HCl accompanied by a ^{44}Ti breakthrough of 90 Bq representing a separation factor of 2×10^6 [31]. Long-term stability of the generator is ensured by a reverse elution mode which is needed to provide high retention of titanium-44 on the column [31]. This concept leads to a generator design providing scandium-44 in stable yields without significant ^{44}Ti-breakthrough since approximate 10 years.

As volume, pH and eluent composition of the 180 MBq ^{44}Ti/^{44}Sc generator are not suitable for subsequent radiolabeling, for example, peptides for clinical application, an efficient post-processing strategy in analogy to the post-processing approach of ^{68}Ge/^{68}Ga generators was developed [40, 64, 65]. This post-processing includes reduction of the volume of ^{44}Sc solution, optimization of pH for subsequent radiolabeling as well as further purification from metal contaminants disturbing the complex formation by utilizing a cation exchange column. Finally, ~ 90% of chemically and radiochemically highly pure scandium-44 can be recovered in 3 ml 0.25 M ammonium acetate (pH = 4) with less than 7 Bq ^{44}Ti-breakthrough within 10 min ready for following radiolabeling reactions [21, 38, 40].

2.2. Synthesis of [^{44}Sc]Sc-PSMA-617

DOTA is used as bifunctional chelator in PSMA-617 (cf. **Figure 1**) requiring elevated temperatures for complex formation. Commonly DOTA-based radiopharmaceuticals are prepared using 95°C; therefore, it was evident to choose this as radiolabeling temperature for generator as well as for cyclotron produced scandium-44 [21, 25].

Due to the low activity obtained from the ^{44}Ti/^{44}Sc-generator, evaluation of the influence of precursor amount and reaction time on radiochemical yield resulted in apparent molar activities of 6.50 ± 0.76 MBq/nmol [21] while values of 5–10 MBq/nmol using cyclotron produced scandium-44 are possible [20].

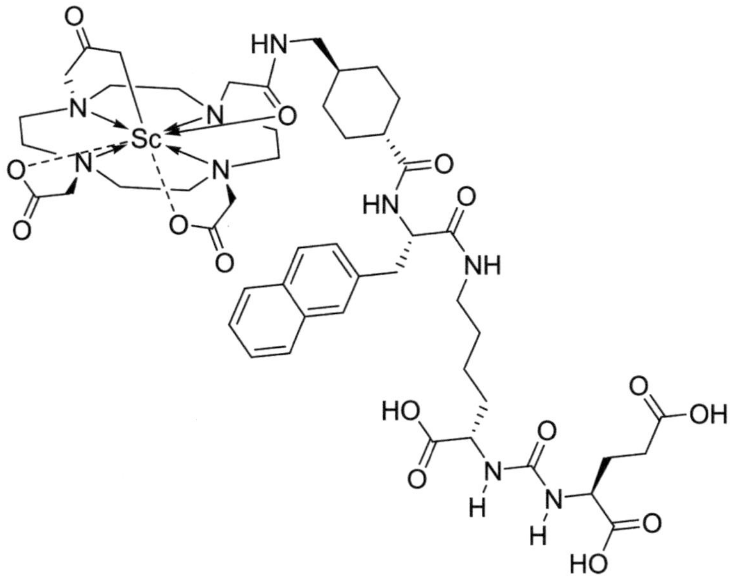

Figure 1. Putative structure of [^{44}Sc]Sc-PSMA-617.

With regard to the reported radiochemical yields of >97% [20, 21], it seems not necessary to evaluate a purification method. Nevertheless, removal of unwanted ions (e.g., acetate ions, uncomplexed $^{44}Sc^{3+}$) from the crude product solution is of interest especially with a view to clinical application. The purification method of choice is solid phase extraction. This cheap and easy method is commonly used when it is necessary to purify radiopharmaceuticals. Solid phase extraction with C-18 cartridges was suitable for further purification. After equilibration of the cartridge, almost quantitative retention of [^{44}Sc]Sc-PSMA-617 on the cartridge and product recovery with >90% efficacy is possible [21].

2.3. Preclinical evaluation

The evaluation of the logD values of the ^{68}Ga-, ^{44}Sc- and ^{177}Lu-complexes and [^{68}Ga]Ga-PSMA-11 revealed that the values are in the same range for the PSMA-617 complexes and reduced for [^{68}Ga]Ga-PSMA-11(cf. **Table 4**) [20].

The presence of metal cations like Fe^{3+} or other chelators can cause a release of the radionuclide from PSMA-617. As this is a crucial factor for later use as a radiopharmaceutical stability of [^{44}Sc]Sc-PSMA-617 against transmetallation, transchelation as well as its stability in human serum and in final formulation was investigated. To determine the stability in the presence of relevant metal cations, those typically present in vivo (Ca^{2+}, Fe^{3+}, Mg^{2+}), at levels significantly higher compared to normal in vivo levels, were chosen. Transchelation was determined against DTPA and EDTA, two chelators forming scandium complexes already at room temperature. In all stability experiments more than 95% of [^{44}Sc]Sc-PSMA-617 remained intact even after 24 h incubation [21]. (cf. **Table 3**).

Eppard et al. as well as Umbricht et al. determined the binding affinity of ^{nat}Sc-PSMA-617 but by different methods and cell lines [20, 21]. Due to the differences in the experimental set up, the results are not directly comparable. Nevertheless, there are similarities. Binding affinity to the target were for [^{44}Sc]Sc-PSMA-617 and [^{177}Lu]Lu-PSMA-617 in the same range cf. (**Table 4**). Similar results could be observed for the internalization of the radioligands. Uptake was comparable for all compounds without any significant differences within the

Time (h)	% intact [^{44}Sc]Sc-PSMA-617 ± SD						
	Ca^{2+}	Mg^{2+}	Fe^{3+}	EDTA	DTPA	NaCl	Human serum
0.5	98.0 ± 0.0	98.7 ± 0.5	97.3 ± 0.9	96.7 ± 0.1	96.7 ± 1.2	98.7 ± 0.5	98.7 ± 0.5
1	98.3 ± 0.5	98.3 ± 0.5	98.0 ± 0.8	97.3 ± 0.1	97.7 ± 0.5	98.0 ± 0–8	98.0 ± 0.8
2	97.0 ± 0.1	98.0 ± 0.8	98.0 ± 0.8	97.3 ± 0.1	97.0 ± 0.8	97.7 ± 1.3	98.0 ± 0.4
4	97.0 ± 1.4	97.7 ± 0.5	96.7 ± 0.5	97.3 ± 0.1	96.7 ± 0.5	97.3 ± 0.5	97.0 ± 0.8
24	96.7 ± 0.8	97.2 ± 0.8	95.0 ± 1.4	95.9 ± 1.2	95.1 ± 0.8	96.0 ± 0.8	96.3 ± 0.9

Table 3. Stability of [^{44}Sc]Sc-PSMA-617 at 37°C in the presence of different metal cations and in the presence of DTPA and EDTA, at 10^{-2} M concentration respectively (n = 3).

	Log D	Relative PSMA-binding affinity	
		LNCaP cells	PC-3 PIP cells
[^{44}Sc]Sc-PSMA-617	−4.21 ± 0.04	1.47	1.18
[^{177}Lu]Lu-PSMA-617	−4.18 ± 0.06	1	1
[^{68}Ga]Ga-PSMA-617	−4.30 ± 0.10	1.08	0.54
[^{68}Ga]Ga-PSMA-11	−4.82 ± 0.07	0.58	0.45

Table 4. Log D (n = 3–5) and relative PSMA-binding affinity as the inverse molar ratio of the average K_D values as determined in cell studies with LNCaP cells [21] and PC-3 PIP cells [20] according to Reddy et al. [66].

experimental set up [20, 21]. Additionally, it was possible to prove PSMA-specific uptake/internalization for all radioligands used employing a PC-3 PIP/flu tumor model [20, 21].

Umbricht et al. performed biodistribution and small animal imaging studies in PC-3 PIP and PC-3 flu tumor-bearing mice directly comparing [^{44}Sc]Sc-PSMA-617 with [^{177}Lu]Lu-PSMA-617, [^{68}Ga]Ga-PSMA-617 and [^{68}Ga]Ga-PSMA-11 under the same in vivo conditions [20]. The study confirmed comparable in vitro behavior, which was expected due to similar coordination behavior of scandium-44 and lutetium-177 [20, 48]. The similar chemical behavior of the two nuclides is also evident in vivo in the pharmacokinetics of the radiopharmaceuticals. [^{44}Sc]Sc-PSMA-617 and [^{177}Lu]Lu-PSMA-617 revealed a largely identical biodistribution within in the investigated period of time [20]. Along with the advantage of the longer half-life of scandium-44, enabling late-time imaging, the increasing tumor-to-background ratio over time can be exploited [20]. Additional comparison with the [^{68}Ga]Ga-PSMA-617 confirmed small differences in the pharmacokinetics of [^{68}Ga]Ga-PSMA-617 and [^{177}Lu]Lu-PSMA-617 explainable with the different coordination chemistry of gallium and lutetium [20].

2.4. Synthesis and quality control for human use

The pharmacopeia contains recognized pharmaceutical rules on the quality, testing, storage and labeling of medicinal products and the substances, materials and methods used in their manufacture and testing. It is legally binding [21].

As scandium-44 is a new isotope for human PET application, there is no monograph in the European or another pharmacopeia available for the preparation of scandium-44 or ^{44}Sc-radiopharmaceuticals. Therefore, quality control was performed based on the monograph for [^{68}Ga]Ga-DOTATOC of the European Pharmacopeia [67].

With respect to the use of generator-derived scandium-44, special attention has to be paid to the quality control of the titanium-44 content in the final formulation.

To ensure the quality of [^{44}Sc]Sc-PSMA-617, the radiolabeling procedure was modified for patient application. Since only a maximum of 180 MBq scandium-44 is available via the generator per elution and the time from the beginning of the generator elution to the injection to the patient is 3–4 h, it was necessary to guarantee high and stable radiochemical yields. To achieve this, the amount of precursor was increased to 38.4 nmol, and 9 vol% ethanol was added to the radiolabeling mixture. Ethanol has two tasks: to improve radiolabeling efficacy [68] and to prevent radiolysis in the initial radiolabeling mixture. Its use as scavenger is very important to ensure radiochemical purity as radiolysis by-products can cause undesired and serious side effects while their removal is time-consuming and complicated. Additionally, C-18 purification was performed by default. This step removes potentially remaining ^{44}Ti-breakthrough, uncomplexed scandium-44 as well as ammonium acetate buffer prior to final formulation of the radiopharmaceutical. Although this step extends synthesis time, its contribution to ensure radiochemical and especially radionuclidic purity is very important. With respect to the use of generator-derived scandiuim-44, the ^{44}Ti-breakthrough was of major interest. During process set-up, it was even tested twice, in the radiolabeling mixture and final formulation. It was measured not earlier than 120 h after synthesis in a γ-spectrometer at 67.9 and 78.3 keV. Titanium-44 was not traceable in any of the quality control samples.

Due to the limited activity derived from the ^{44}Ti/^{44}Sc-generator system, the apparent molar activity was 3.05 ± 0.36 MBq/nmol at time of calibration (end of synthesis) which is considerably lower compared to [^{68}Ga]Ga-PSMA-11 (14–355 MBq/nmol) or [^{68}Ga]Ga-DOTA-TOC (4–72 MBq/nmol).

Parameters checked during the quality control procedure were listed in **Table 5**.

Due to the nature of radiopharmaceuticals sterility, breakthrough and content of long living radionuclides could not be determined before release of the final radiopharmaceutical. Therefore, only a preliminary release was possible. Final release of the respective batch was performed with receipt of the last test results.

	Method	Acceptance criteria
Volume activity	Dose calibrator	5–15 MBq/ml
Visual appearance	Optical	Clear, colorless
Drug Identity	Radio-HPLC	11.3 ± 0.4 min
Nuclide identity	γ-Spectroscopy	511 ± 25 keV
	Decay measurements	3.97 ± 0.2 h
pH	Indicator strip	4–8.5
Apparent molar activity	Calculation	0.7–8 MBq/nmol
Radiochemical purity	Radio-HPLC/Radio-TLC	≥ 95%
Long living nuclides	γ-Spectroscopy	Yes/No
Breakthrough	γ-Spectroscopy	< 0.001%
Filter integrity	Bubble point	> 3447 mbar
Endotoxins	LAL-test	< 17.5 IU/ml
Sterility	According Ph. Eur.	Sterile

Table 5. Parameters checked during quality control with acceptance criteria and average value measured.

3. Part II: Dosimetry

Theranostics and personalized medicine in oncology are in need for highly sensitive and specific diagnostic PET probes that may be radiolabeled with therapeutic radionuclides [18]. It is assumed that diagnostic PET agent distribution is more appropriate for prediction of therapeutic dose increasing therapeutic outcome [18]. Among the several matched pairs for imaging and therapy used in nuclear medicine, focus is on the PET nuclides gallium-68 and scandium-44 as imaging counterpart for lutetium-177.

3.1. Methodology

For the first clinical application, five men with progressive mCRPC enrolled for [^{177}Lu]Lu-PSMA-617 therapy received [^{44}Sc]Sc-PSMA-617 for PET imaging (cf. **Table 6**) [21, 69, 70].

The study protocol stipulates PET/CT imaging starting with a dynamic PET scan of abdomen with kidneys in the field of view (FOV) followed by a low dose CT scan and three static whole-body scans from skull to mid-thigh acquired 45 minutes, 2 h and 19.5 h post injection with preceding low-dose CT. Quantitative analysis was performed visually to identify organs of increased tracer uptake as source organs for further dosimetric calculations. Residence times, organ-absorbed doses (mSv/MBq) as well as effective doses were calculated during quantitative analysis [21, 69, 70] and the maximum permissible activity as well as the maximum number of therapy cycles (6 GBq per cycle) which can be administered were determined [70].

3.2. First in-human studies

Following the promising preclinical results, Eppard et al. conducted a first-in-human application [21, 69, 70].

In all patients, PSMA-positive metastases were detectable by [^{44}Sc]Sc-PSMA-617 PET/CT applying a single dose of 50.45 ± 9.25 MBq. Visual comparison with images from previous [^{68}Ga]Ga-PSMA-11-PET/CT those from [^{44}Sc]Sc-PSMA-617 PET/CT were found to

Patient no.	Age	Weight (kg)	Hematocrit	Injected activity (MBq)	Injected activity (MBq/kg)	PSA (ng/ml)
1	70	78	0.33	50.00	0.64	453.00
2	72	80	0.30	62.23	0.78	26.00
3	67	70	0.39	39.61	0.57	7.20
4	70	80	0.30	50.00	0.63	139.00
5	67	104	0.29	48.95	0.47	3000.0
Mean	69	82.4	0.32	50.16	0.62	
SD	2.2	12.76	0.04	8.04	0.11	

Table 6. Details of study population [21, 69, 70].

be at least equal at a significantly reduced dose. Direct comparison of [^{68}Ga]Ga-PSMA-11 and [^{44}Sc]Sc-PSMA-617 PET/CT images as well as planar scintigraphy and SPECT/CT of [^{177}Lu]Lu-PSMA-617 in one patient is depicted in **Figure 2**.

Due to the longer half-life of scandium-44, patient management could become more flexible through its use allowing PET/CT imaging several hours post injection (**Figure 3**) [20]. Indeed using low doses still and late time point imaging still enables detection of lesions while accumulated activity in urinary tract or kidney is no longer observed [21]. Qualitative detection of PSMA-positive lesions is feasible due to increased tumor-to-background ratios and resulting improved image contrast [21].

Khawar et al. reported estimated residence times (MBq-h/MBq) to be prolonged in the liver followed by the kidneys, urinary bladder, bone marrow and rest of organs compared with [^{68}Ga]Ga-PSMA-617 [69]. Also, the study revealed that kidneys (3.19E-01 mSv/MBq;

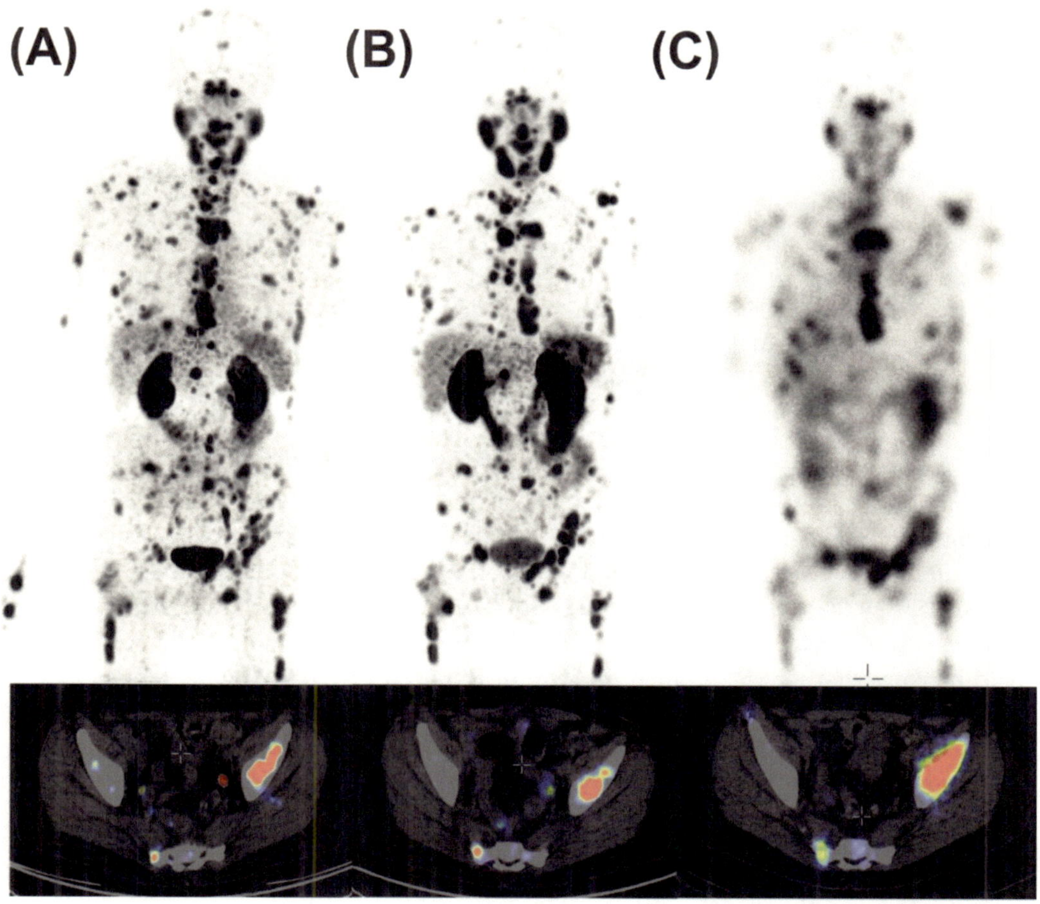

Figure 2. Maximal intensity projection (top) and representative slice (bottom) of PET/CT examination of a 70-year-old patient suffering of mCRPC with high tumor load using (A) [^{44}Sc]Sc-PSMA-617 (50 MBq, 60 min p.i.), and (B) [^{68}Ga]Ga-PSMA-11 (120 MBq, 60 min p.i.). (C) On the right-hand side, the planar scintigraphy (top) and a representative slice of the post-therapy SPECT/CT scan, about 24 h after application of 6.7 GBq of [^{177}Lu]Lu-PSMA-617 are shown [21].

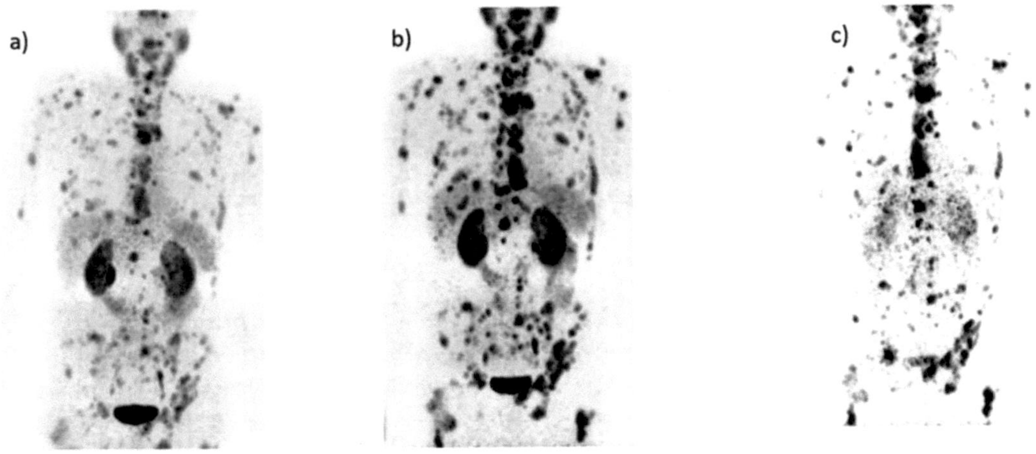

Figure 3. PET/CT whole body images at different time points p.i. using [^{44}Sc]Sc-PSMA-617: (A) 30 min, (B) 120 min, and (C) 19 h [21].

range: 1.78 E-01-4.88E-01 mSv/MBq) are the critical organs at risk receiving the highest dose followed by the urinary bladder wall, spleen, salivary glands, liver and small intestine while bone marrow dose was less and consequently not included in organs at risk for therapeutic application [69]. These findings are consistent with the results for small PSMA ligands of previous studies [71, 72]. Overall, the study confirmed absorbed doses to be higher for [^{44}Sc]Sc-PSMA-617 than for [^{68}Ga]Ga-PSMA-617, [^{68}Ga]Ga-PSMA-11, [^{68}Ga]Ga-PSMA-I&T but less than [^{124}I]I-PSMA [69]. Also the mean effective dose was found to be higher than [^{68}Ga]Ga-PSMA-617, [^{68}Ga]Ga-PSMA-11, [^{68}Ga]Ga-PSMA-I&T but less than [^{124}I]I-PSMA [69, 72].

In a follow-up study, Khawar et al. used [^{44}Sc]Sc-PSMA-617 PET/CT for pre-therapeutic dosimetry estimating the organ doses of [^{177}Lu]Lu-PSMA-617 administered [70]. This was performed by mathematical exploration of pharmacokinetics of [^{44}Sc]Sc-PSMA-617 to that of [^{177}Lu]Lu-PSMA-617. As preclinical in vitro and in vivo studies proofed better correlation between [^{44}Sc]Sc-PSMA-617 and [^{177}Lu]Lu-PSMA-617 as compared to ^{68}Ga-PSMA agents, the authors assumed that dosimetric analysis from 19.5 h imaging data of [^{44}Sc]Sc-PSMA-617 could be converted into 6.7 d imaging data for [^{177}Lu]Lu-PSMA-617 [20, 70]. Total activity (MBq) in source organs and whole body from reconstructed images of dynamic data, and three static whole body PET/CT images were decay corrected back to time of injection using scandium-44 half-life and then forward decay corrected using half-life of lutetium-177 for calculation [70].

Table 7 shows the mean residence times (MBq-h/MBq) for [^{44}Sc]Sc-PSMA-617 and based on [^{44}Sc]Sc-PSMA-617 pharmacokinetics for [^{177}Lu]Lu-PSMA-617 [69, 70].

Also for [^{177}Lu]Lu-PSMA-617, kidneys appeared to be the organ at risk (mean absorbed dose 0.44 mSv/MBq) followed by the salivary glands, liver, small intestine, spleen and urinary bladder wall [70]. The mean bone marrow absorbed dose was reported to be 0.05 mSv/MBq,

PT No	[44Sc]Sc-PSMA-617		[177Lu]Lu-PSMA-617	
	Mean±	SD	Mean±	SD
Organs				
Salivary glands	0.03±	0.027	0.24	0.21
Kidneys	0.24±	0.109	1.51	0.48
Liver	0.35±	0.263	4.46	1.72
Spleen	0.07±	0.031	0.18	0.07
Small Intestine	0.05±	0.029	0.63	0.37
Bone marrow	0.09±	0.047	0.52	0.69
Urinary bladder contents	0.18±	0.195	0.33	0.32
Remainder of body	1.82	0.684	46.58	16.04

Table 7. Mean residence times (MBq-h/MBq) fcr [44Sc]Sc-PSMA-617 and estimated for [177Lu]Lu-PSMA-617 on basis of [44Sc]Sc-PSMA-617 pharmacokinetics [69, 70].

and the mean whole body dose was 0.08 mSv/MBq [70]. These findings are comparable with literature [11, 13, 17, 19]. Total dose (Gy) per cycle administered lies in a range from 2 till 3.26 Gy although applying the same therapeutic activities [70]. Due to the use of 3D instead of usual 2 D dosimetric analysis, it was found that it is possible to administer a mean dose of 52 Gy to reach a dose limit of 23 Gy [70] which is significantly higher than reported before with 30 Gy [13].

All together both studies proved that dosimetry using [44Sc]Sc-PSMA-617 PET/CT is possible applying a protocol which could be implemented in clinical daily routine.

4. Conclusion

Recent studies demonstrated the high potential of [44Sc]Sc-PSMA-617 for PET imaging in a preclinical as well as a clinical setting where it revealed more similar characteristics to [177Lu]Lu-PSMA-617 than the routinely used [68Ga]Ga-PSMA-11 [20, 21].

While images at early time points are comparable with those of [68Ga]Ga-PSMA-11, the advantages of scandium-44 over gallium-68 show up at late time points due to its longer half-life. Enabling delayed image acquisition would simplify patient management at improved image quality and allows improved pre-therapeutic dosimetry for therapy with [177Lu]Lu-PSMA-617. Especially for pre-therapeutic dosimetry scandium-44 would be beneficial as implementation in the clinical setting is uncomplicated, and there is no need for patient hospitalization. Together with the possibility transporting scandium-44 and ^{44}Sc-radiopharmaceuticals further routes to radiopharmaceutical institutions without option for in-house production scandium-44 could make a significant contribution to patient care even in remote areas.

Author details

Elisabeth Eppard

Address all correspondence to: e.eppard@web.de

Johannes Gutenberg-University Mainz, Mainz, Germany

References

[1] UNPB. World Health Organization. International Agency for Research on Cancer. May 15, 2018. http://gco.iarc.fr/today/fact-sheets-cancers?cancer=19&type=0&sex=1

[2] Ahmadzadehfar H, Eppard E, Kürpig S, Fimmers R, Yordanova A, Schlenkhoff CD, et al. Therapeutic response and side effects of repeated radioligand therapy with 177Lu-PSMA-DKFZ-617 of castrate-resistant metastatic prostate cancer. Oncotarget. 2016;**7**:12477-12488. DOI: 10.18632/oncotarget.7245

[3] Rahbar K, Ahmadzadehfar H, Kratochwil C, Haberkorn U, Schäfers M, Essler M, et al. German Multicenter study investigating 177Lu-PSMA-617 Radioligand therapy in advanced prostate Cancer patients. Journal of Nuclear Medicine. 2017;**58**:85-90. DOI: 10.2967/jnumed.116.183194

[4] Ghosh A, Heston WDW. Tumor target prostate specific membrane antigen (PSMA) and its regulation in prostate cancer. Journal of Cellular Biochemistry. 2004;**91**:528-539. DOI: 10.1002/jcb.10661

[5] Ahmadzadehfar H. Targeted therapy for metastatic prostate cancer with radionuclides. In: Mohan R, editor. Prostate Cancer - Leading-Edge Diagnostic Procedures and Treatments. Croatia: InTech; 2016. DOI: 10.5772/64016

[6] Pfestroff A, Luster M, Jilg CA, Olbert PJ, Ohlmann CH, Lassmann M, et al. Current status and future perspectives of PSMA-targeted therapy in Europe: Opportunity knocks. European Journal of Nuclear Medicine and Molecular Imaging. 2015;**42**:1971-1975. DOI: 10.1007/s00259-015-3186-3

[7] Benesova M, Schafer M, Bauder-Wust U, Afshar-Oromieh A, Kratochwil C, Mier W, et al. Preclinical evaluation of a tailor-made DOTA-conjugated PSMA inhibitor with optimized linker moiety for imaging and Endoradiotherapy of prostate Cancer. Journal of Nuclear Medicine. 2015;**56**:914-920. DOI: 10.2967/jnumed.114.147413

[8] Ahmadzadehfar H, Wegen S, Yordanova A, Fimmers R, Kurpig S, Eppard E, et al. Overall survival and response pattern of castration-resistant metastatic prostate cancer to multiple cycles of radioligand therapy using 177LuLu-PSMA-617. European Journal of Nuclear Medicine and Molecular Imaging. 2017;**44**:1448-1454. DOI: 10.1007/s00259-017-3716-2

[9] Ahmadzadehfar H, Rahbar K, Kurpig S, Bogemann M, Claesener M, Eppard E, et al. Early side effects and first results of radioligand therapy with (177)Lu-DKFZ-617 PSMA

of castrate-resistant metastatic prostate cancer: A two-Centre study. EJNMMI Research. 2015;**5**:114. DOI: 10.1186/s13550-015-0114-2

[10] Yordanova A, Becker A, Eppard E, Kurpig S, Fisang C, Feldmann G, et al. The impact of repeated cycles of radioligand therapy using 177LuLu-PSMA-617 on renal function in patients with hormone refractory metastatic prostate cancer. European Journal of Nuclear Medicine and Molecular Imaging. 2017;**44**:1473-1479. DOI: 10.1007/s00259-017-3681-9

[11] Fendler WP, Reinhardt S, Ilhan H, Delker A, Böning G, Gildehaus FJ, et al. Preliminary experience with dosimetry, response and patient reported outcome after 177Lu-PSMA-617 therapy for metastatic castration-resistant prostate cancer. Oncotarget. 2017;**8**:3581-3590. DOI: 10.18632/oncotarget.12240

[12] Baum RP, Kulkarni HR, Schuchardt C, Singh A, Wirtz M, Wiessalla S, et al. 177Lu-Labeled prostate-specific membrane antigen Radioligand therapy of metastatic castration-resistant prostate Cancer: Safety and efficacy. Journal of Nuclear Medicine. 2016;**57**:1006-1013. DOI: 10.2967/jnumed.115.168443

[13] Delker A, Fendler WP, Kratochwil C, Brunegraf A, Gosewisch A, Gildehaus FJ, et al. Dosimetry for (177)Lu-DKFZ-PSMA-617: A new radiopharmaceutical for the treatment of metastatic prostate cancer. European Journal of Nuclear Medicine and Molecular Imaging. 2016;**43**:42-51. DOI: 10.1007/s00259-015-3174-7

[14] Kabasakal L, AbuQbeitah M, Aygun A, Yeyin N, Ocak M, Demirci E, Toklu T. Pre-therapeutic dosimetry of normal organs and tissues of (177)Lu-PSMA-617 prostate-specific membrane antigen (PSMA) inhibitor in patients with castration-resistant prostate cancer. European Journal of Nuclear Medicine and Molecular Imaging. 2015;**42**:1976-1983. DOI: 10.1007/s00259-015-3125-3

[15] Rahbar K, Schmidt M, Heinzel A, Eppard E, Bode A, Yordanova A, et al. Response and tolerability of a single dose of 177Lu-PSMA-617 in patients with metastatic castration-resistant prostate Cancer: A Multicenter retrospective analysis. Journal of Nuclear Medicine. 2016;**57**:1334-1338. DOI: 10.2967/jnumed.116.173757

[16] Zechmann CM, Afshar-Oromieh A, Armor T, Stubbs JB, Mier W, Hadaschik B, et al. Radiation dosimetry and first therapy results with a (124)I/ (131)I-labeled small molecule (MIP-1095) targeting PSMA for prostate cancer therapy. European Journal of Nuclear Medicine and Molecular Imaging. 2014;**41**:1280-1292. DOI: 10.1007/s00259-014-2713-y

[17] Kratochwil C, Giesel FL, Stefanova M, Benešová M, Bronzel M, Afshar-Oromieh A, et al. PSMA-targeted radionuclide therapy of metastatic castration-resistant prostate Cancer with 177Lu-Labeled PSMA-617. Journal of Nuclear Medicine. 2016;**57**:1170-1176. DOI: 10.2967/jnumed.115.171397

[18] Kulkarni HR, Singh A, Schuchardt C, Niepsch K, Sayeg M, Leshch Y, et al. PSMA-based radioligand therapy for metastatic castration-resistant prostate cancer: The bad Berka experience since 2013. Journal of Nuclear Medicine. 2016;**57**:97S-104S. DOI: 10.2967/jnumed.115.170167

[19] Okamoto S, Thieme A, Allmann J, D'Alessandria C, Maurer T, Retz M, et al. Radiation dosimetry for 177Lu-PSMA I&T in metastatic castration-resistant prostate cancer: Absorbed dose in normal organs and tumor lesions. Journal of Nuclear Medicine. 2017;**58**:445-450. DOI: 10.2967/jnumed.116.178483

[20] Umbricht CA, Benesova M, Schmid RM, Turler A, Schibli R, van der Meulen, Nicholas P, Muller C. 44Sc-PSMA-617 for radiotheragnostics in tandem with 177Lu-PSMA-617-preclinical investigations in comparison with 68Ga-PSMA-11 and 68Ga-PSMA-617. EJNMMI Research. 2017;**7**:9. DOI: 10.1186/s13550-017-0257-4

[21] Eppard E, de La FA, Benešová M, Khawar A, Bundschuh RA, Gärtner FC, et al. Clinical translation and first in-human use of 44ScSc-PSMA-617 for PET imaging of metastasized castrate-resistant prostate cancer. Theranostics. 2017;**7**:4359-4369. DOI: 10.7150/thno.20586

[22] Schäfer M, Bauder-Wüst U, Leotta K, Zoller F, Mier W, Haberkorn U, et al. A dimerized urea-based inhibitor of the prostate-specific membrane antigen for 68Ga-PET imaging of prostate cancer. European Journal of Nuclear Medicine and Molecular Imaging Research. 2012;**2**:23

[23] Eder M, Schäfer M, Bauder-Wüst U, Hull W-E, Wängler C, Mier W, et al. 68 Ga-complex lipophilicity and the targeting property of a urea-based PSMA inhibitor for PET imaging. Bioconjugate Chemistry. 2012;**23**:688-697. DOI: 10.1021/bc200279b

[24] http://www.nndc.bnl.gov/chart. [Accessed: 16 May 2018]

[25] Domnanich KA, Müller C, Farkas R, Schmid RM, Ponsard B, Schibli R, et al. 44Sc for labeling of DOTA- and NODAGA-functionalized peptides: Preclinical in vitro and in vivo investigations. EJNMMI Radiopharmacy and Chemistry. 2017;**1**:2. DOI: 10.1186/s41181-016-0013-5

[26] Hernandez R, Valdovinos HF, Yang Y, Chakravarty R, Hong H, Barnhart TE, Cai W. (44)Sc: An attractive isotope for peptide-based PET imaging. Molecular Pharmaceutics. 2014;**11**:2954-2961. DOI: 10.1021/mp500343j

[27] Muller C, Bunka M, Reber J, Fischer C, Zhernosekov K, Turler A, Schibli R. Promises of cyclotron-produced 44Sc as a diagnostic match for trivalent beta--emitters: In vitro and in vivo study of a 44Sc-DOTA-folate conjugate. Journal of Nuclear Medicine. 2013;**54**:2168-2174. DOI: 10.2967/jnumed.113.123810

[28] Müller C, Bunka M, Haller S, Köster U, Groehn V, Bernhardt P, et al. Promising prospects for 44Sc-/47Sc-based theragnostics: Application of 47Sc for radionuclide tumor therapy in mice. Journal of Nuclear Medicine. 2014;**55**:1658-1664. DOI: 10.2967/jnumed.114.141614

[29] Singh A, Baum RP, Klette I, van der Meulen, Nicholas P, Muller C, Tuerler A, Schibli R. Scandium-44 DOTATOC PET/CT: First in-human molecular imaging of neuroendocrine tumors and possible perspectives for Theranostics. Journal of Nuclear Medicine 2015;**56**:267

[30] Rösch F. Scandium-44: Benefits of a long-lived PET radionuclides available from the 44Ti/44Sc generator system. Current Radiopharmaceuticals. 2012;**5**:187-201

[31] Filosofov DV, Loktionova NS, Rösch F. A 44Ti/44Sc radionuclide generator for potential application of 44Sc-based PET-radiopharmaceuticals. Radiochimica Acta. 2010;**98**:149-156

[32] Greene MW, Hillman M. A scandium generator. The International Journal of Applied Radiation and Isotopes. 1967;**18**:540-541

[33] Alliot C, Kerdjoudj R, Michel N, Haddad F, Huclier-Markai S. Cyclotron production of high purity (44m,44)Sc with deuterons from (44)CaCO3 targets. Nuclear Medicine and Biology. 2015;**42**:524-529. DOI: 10.1016/j.nucmedbio.2015.03.002

[34] Wittwer D, Dressler R, Eichler R, Gäggeler HW, Piguet D, Serov A, et al. The thermal release of scandium from titanium metal – A simple way to produce pure 44 Sc for PET application. Radiochimica Acta. 2011;**99**:193-196. DOI: 10.1524/ract.2011.1832

[35] Seidl E, Lieser KH. Die Radionuklidgeneratoren 113Sn/113mIn, 68Ge/68Ga und 44Ti/44Sc. Radiochimica Acta. 1973;**19**:196-199

[36] Radchenko V, Meyer CAL, Engle JW, Naranjo CM, Unc GA, Mastren T, et al. Separation of 44Ti from proton irradiated scandium by using solid-phase extraction chromatography and design of 44Ti/44Sc generator system. Journal of Chromatography. A. 2016;**1477**: 39-46

[37] Rösch F, Baum RP. Generator-based PET radiopharmaceuticals for molecular imaging of tumours: On the way to THERANOSTICS. Dalton Transactions. 2011;**40**:6104-6111. DOI: 10.1039/c0dt01398f

[38] Pruszyński M, Majkowska-Pilip A, Loktionova NS, Eppard E, Roesch F. Radiolabeling of DOTATOC with the long-lived positron emitter 44Sc. Applied Radiation and Isotopes. 2012;**70**:974-979. DOI: 10.1016/j.apradiso.2012.03.005

[39] Alenitzky YG, Novgorodov AF, Filosofov DV, Skripnik AV, Kaplun VG, Suzikov AG, Eliseev IA, Rösch F. ^{44}Ti: Investigation of Target Preparation, Irradiation and Yields in the 45Sc(p,2n) Process. Mainz; 2005. E:\1 - Bibliothek\Paper\2005 Jahresberich KC MZ.pdf

[40] Pruszynski M, Loktionova NS, Filosofov DV, Rösch F. Post-elution processing of 44Ti/44Sc generator-derived 44Sc for clinical application. Applied Radiation and Isotopes. 2010;**68**:1636-1641. DOI: 10.1016/j.apradiso.2010.04.003

[41] Nagy G, Szikra D, Trencsényi G, Fekete A, Garai I, Giani AM, et al. AAZTA: An ideal chelating agent for the development of 44 Sc PET imaging agents. Angewandte Chemie. 2017;**129**:2150-2154. DOI: 10.1002/ange.201611207

[42] Mausner LF, Joshi V, Kolsky KL, Meinken GE, Mease RC, Sweet MP, Srivastava SC. Evaluation of chelating agents for radioimmunotherapy with scandium-47. Journal of Nuclear Medicine. 1995;**36**:104

[43] Koumarianou E, Loktionova NS, Fellner M, Roesch F, Thews O, Pawlak D, et al. 44Sc-DOTA-BN[2-14]NH2 in comparison to 68Ga-DOTA-BN[2-14]NH2 in pre-clinical investigation. Is 44Sc a potential radionuclide for PET? Applied Radiation and Isotopes. 2012;**70**:2669-2676. DOI: 10.1016/j.apradiso.2012.08.004

[44] Anderson WT, Strand M. Stability, targeting, and biodistribution of scandium-46- and gallium-67-labeled monoclonal antibody in erythroleukemic mice. PubMed - NCBI. https://

www.ncbi.nlm.nih.gov/pubmed/?term=Cancer+Res.+45+(1985)+2154%E2%80%932158. [Accessed: 7 May 2018]

[45] Cotton SA. Recent advances in the chemistry of scandium. Polyhedron. 1999;**18**:1691-1715. DOI: 10.1016/S0277-5387(99)00039-X

[46] Meehan PR, Aris DR, Willey GR. Structural chemistry of Sc(III): An overview. Coordination Chemistry Reviews. 1999;**181**:121-145. DOI: 10.1016/S0010-8545(98)00214-8

[47] Marques F, Gano L, Paula Campello M, Lacerda S, Santos I, Lima LMP, et al. 13- and 14-membered macrocyclic ligands containing methylcarboxylate or methylphosphonate pendant arms: Chemical and biological evaluation of their (153)Sm and (166)Ho complexes as potential agents for therapy or bone pain palliation. Journal of Inorganic Biochemistry. 2006;**100**:270-280. DOI: 10.1016/j.jinorgbio.2005.11.011

[48] Majkowska-Pilip A, Bilewicz A. Macrocyclic complexes of scandium radionuclides as precursors for diagnostic and therapeutic radiopharmaceuticals. Journal of Inorganic Biochemistry. 2011;**105**:313-320

[49] Zhernosekov K, Bunka M, Hohn A, Schibli R, Türler A. Development and evaluation of (44)Ti production on high energy protons. Journal of Labelled Compounds and Radiopharmaceuticals 2011;**54**:S239. DOIL 10.1002/jlcr.1926

[50] Duchemin C, Guertin A, Haddad F, Michel N, Métivier V. Production of scandium-44 m and scandium-44 g with deuterons on calcium-44: Cross section measurements and production yield calculations. Physics in Medicine and Biology. 2015;**60**:6847-6864. DOI: 10.1088/0031-9155/60/17/6847

[51] Kamel A, Cydzik I, Federica S, Krajewski S, Kasparek A, Bilewics A. Cyclotron production of 44Sc - new radionuclide for PET technique. Journal of Labelled Compounds and Radiopharmaceuticals. 2011;**54**. DOI: S53. DOI:10.1002/jlcr.1925

[52] Krajewski S, Cydzik I, Kamel A, Bulgheroni A, Simonell F, Majakowska-Pilip A, Bilewicz A. Simple procedure of dotatate labelling with cyclotron produced 44SC and 43SC. Nuclear Medicine Review. 2012;**15**:22-46

[53] Severin GW, Engle JW, Valdovinos HF, Barnhart TE, Nickles RJ. Cyclotron produced 44gSc from natural calcium. Applied Radiation and Isotopes. 2012;**70**:1526-1530. DOI: 10.1016/j.apradiso.2012.04.030

[54] Szkliniarz K, Sitarz M, Walczak R, Jastrzębski J, Bilewicz A, Choiński J, et al. Production of medical Sc radioisotopes with an alpha particle beam. Applied Radiation and Isotopes. 2016;**118**:182-189. DOI: 10.1016/j.apradiso.2016.07.001

[55] Valdovinos HF, Hernandez R, Barnhart TE, Graves S, Cai W, Nickles RJ. Separation of cyclotron-produced 44Sc from a natural calcium target using a dipentyl pentylphosphonate functionalized extraction resin. Applied Radiation and Isotopes. 2015;**95**:23-29. DOI: 10.1016/j.apradiso.2014.09.020

[56] van der Meulen NP, Bunka M, Domnanich KA, Müller C, Haller S, Vermeulen C, et al. Cyclotron production of (44)Sc: From bench to bedside. Nuclear Medicine and Biology. 2015;**42**:745-751. DOI: 10.1016/j.nucmedbio.2015.05.005

[57] Walczak R, Krajewski S, Szkliniarz K, Sitarz M, Abbas K, Choiński J, et al. Cyclotron production of (43)Sc for PET imaging. EJNMMI Physics. 2015;**2**:33. DOI: 10.1186/s40658-015-0136-x

[58] Hassan HE, Al-Abyad M, Mohamed G. Production of 44Ti→44Sc generator in comparison with direct routes by cyclotrons: Cross section evaluation using nuclear models codes. Arab Journal of Nuclear Sciences and Applications. 2018;**51**

[59] Krajewski S, Cydzik I, Abbas K, Bulgheroni A, Simonelli F, Holzwarth U, Bilewicz A. Cyclotron production of 44 Sc for clinical application. Radiochimica Acta. 2013;**101**:333-338. DOI: 10.1524/ract.2013.2032

[60] Hashimoto T, Nakai K, Wakasaya Y, Tanihata I, Fulop Z, Kumagai H, et al. Half-life of Ti. Nuclear Physics A. 2001;**686**:591-599. DOI: 10.1016/S0375-9474(00)00566-2

[61] Hosain F, Syed I, Spencer RP. The Role of Positron Emitters in Nuclear Medicine with Special Reference to Scandium 44; 1977

[62] Mirza MY, Aziz A. A scandium generator. Radiochimica Acta. 1969;**11**:43-44

[63] Radchenko V, Engle JW, Medvedev DG, Maassen JM, Naranjo CM, Unc GA, et al. Proton-induced production and radiochemical isolation of 44Ti from scandium metal targets for 44Ti/44Sc generator development. Nuclear Medicine and Biology. 2017;**50**:25-32. DOI: 10.1016/j.nucmedbio.2017.03.006

[64] Asti M, Gd P, Fraternali A, Grassi E, Sghedoni R, Fioroni F, et al. Validation of 68Ge/68Ga generator processing by chemical purification for routine clinical application of 68Ga-DOTATOC. Nuclear Medicine and Biology. 2008;**35**:721-724. DOI: 10.1016/j.nucmedbio.2008.04.006

[65] Zhernosekov KP, Filosofov DV, Baum RP, Aschoff P, Bihl H, Razbash AA, et al. Processing of generator-produced 68Ga for medical application. Journal of Nuclear Medicine. 2007;**48**:1741-1748

[66] Reddy JA, Xu L-C, Parker N, Vetzel M, Leamon CP. Preclinical evaluation of (99m)Tc-EC20 for imaging folate receptor-positive tumors. Journal of Nuclear Medicine. 2004;**45**:857-866

[67] European Pharmacopoeia: 8.6 to 8.8. Strasbourg: Council Of Europe; 2015

[68] Eppard E, Pèrez-Malo M, Rösch F. Improved radiolabeling of DOTATOC with trivalent radiometals for clinical application by addition of ethanol. EJNMMI Radiopharmacy and Chemistry. 2017;**1**:314. DOI: 10.1186/s41181-016-0010-8

[69] Khawar A, Eppard E, Sinnes JP, Roesch F, Ahmadzadehfar H, Kürpig S, et al. 44ScSc-PSMA-617 biodistribution and dosimetry in patients with metastatic castration-resistant prostate carcinoma. Clinical Nuclear Medicine. 2018;**43**:323-330. DOI: 10.1097/RLU.0000000000002003

[70] Khawar A, Eppard E, Sinnes JP, Roesch F, Ahmadzadehfar H, Kürpig S, et al. Prediction of normal organ absorbed doses for 177LuLu-PSMA-617 using 44ScSc-PSMA-617 pharmacokinetics in patients with metastatic castration resistant prostate carcinoma. Clinical Nuclear Medicine. 2018. DOI: 10.1097/RLU.0000000000002102

[71] Afshar-Oromieh A, Hetzheim H, Kratochwil C, Benesova M, Eder M, Neels OC, et al. The theranostic PSMA ligand PSMA-617 in the diagnosis of prostate cancer by PET/CT: Biodistribution in humans, radiation dosimetry, and first evaluation of tumor lesions. Journal of Nuclear Medicine. 2015;**56**:1697-1705. DOI: 10.2967/jnumed.115.161299

[72] Pfob CH, Ziegler S, Graner FP, Köhner M, Schachoff S, Blechert B, et al. Biodistribution and radiation dosimetry of (68)Ga-PSMA HBED CC-a PSMA specific probe for PET imaging of prostate cancer. European Journal of Nuclear Medicine and Molecular Imaging. 2016;**43**:1962-1970. DOI: 10.1007/s00259-016-3424-3

Section 4

Simple Prostatectomy Technique - Bipolar Endoscopic Prostate Enucleation

Chapter 4

Bipolar Endoscopic Enucleation of Big Benign Prostate Enlargement

Wai Hee Steve Chan, Chi Fai Kan and
Churk Fai Trevor Li

Additional information is available at the end of the chapter

http://dx.doi.org/10.5772/intechopen.79125

Abstract

Large benign prostatic enlargement (BPE) has been a major health problem and the surgical management could be technically challenging to urologists due to the limitation of conventional monopolar transurethral resection of prostate. Bipolar endoscopic enucleation of prostate aimed to remove the adenoma of BPE by stepwise adenoma devascularization and maximal adenoma removal through minimally invasive surgery. In this chapter we described the general principle, the surgical techniques of bipolar endoscopic enucleation and the related modifications of the technique in the recent years. As compared with open prostatectomy, bipolar endoscopic enucleation avoided the wound complications but achieved similar functional outcome. Bipolar endoscopic enucleation also allowed much more adenoma removal comparing with transurethral resection of the prostate. Unlike Holmium laser or thulium laser enucleation of the prostate, the required instruments for bipolar endoscopic enucleation of the prostate were familiar and more readily available to most urologists.

Keywords: benign prostatic hyperplasia, bipolar, enucleation, plasmakinetic, transurethral surgery

1. Introduction

Benign prostatic hyperplasia (BPH) has been a common and important health condition in the modern society. With the aging population, benign prostatic obstruction (BPO) can affect the patients with different degree of bothersome lower urinary tract symptoms or the associated complications. Transurethral resection of the prostate has been the gold standard treatment for benign prostatic obstruction (BPO) with prostate volume 30–80 gm [1]. However, despite its minimally invasive nature and more advanced endoscopes, large benign prostatic enlargement especially over 80 gm remains challenging to urologists due to the increased morbidities related to glycine over-absorption during prolonged operation and transurethral resection of the prostate can resect up to 30–53% of the prostate volume only, leading to problems related to inadequate resection e.g. persistent retention of urine in retention patients and recurrent symptoms [1, 2]. Open prostatectomy provides effective treatment for prostate glands larger than 80 gm through more thorough adenoma removal but yet being most invasive comparing the currently available endoscopic enucleation treatment [1, 3]. However, there were associated problems like wound related complications, prolonged post-operative catheterization and risks of severe hemorrhage [3–6].

Hiraoka described the first endoscopic enucleation of the prostate through monopolar current system in 1983 [7]. However not until the development of model endoscopy system, Holmium:YAG laser, bipolar plasmakinetic system and morcellator, endoscopic enucleation was popularized in the urology field [8]. Gilling reported the technique and outcome of Holmium laser enucleation of the prostate in 1998 [9] but the technique has not been widely adopted due to the learning curve of the procedure and the requirement of high-powered Holmium:YAG laser generator and morcellator.

With the development of bipolar plasmakinetic system in transurethral surgery, transurethral resection can be performed with normal saline irrigation with provides better patient safety and comparable outcome with monopolar system [1]. Neill described the result of his randomized controlled result comparing plasmakinetic enucleation of the prostate with Holmium laser enucleation with Gilling's group in 2006 [9]. Bipolar endoscopic enucleation of prostate is further popularized by Prof Liu CX's group [10] which presented their experience in 1100 patients in 2003–2009, using the technique with only the bipolar transurethral surgery system without the use of morcellator. In the last 15 years, bipolar endoscopic enucleation of the prostate has been reported in many centers with different bipolar transurethral systems, electrodes, modified resection devices and tissue removal technique [3–8, 10–21], so that there was no single unified terminology to describe this technique. In this chapter the term "bipolar endoscopic enucleation of prostate" [12] is used to highlight to key component of this transurethral technique [10–15] and to concur with the term "endoscopic enucleation of the prostate" used in the current guideline in European Association of Urology [1].

2. Surgical technique of bipolar endoscopic enucleation of prostate

2.1. Patient preparation

The indications of bipolar endoscopic enucleation of prostate follow the principle of benign prostate enlargement treatment [1]. The patient would have pre-operative urine culture be performed and treated accordingly to prevent peri-operative urosepsis [22]. Transrectal ultrasound of prostate is recommended in addition to a regular digital rectal examination to evaluate the size of the prostate to avoid prostate size underestimation and the operating surgeons can have a mental image about the shape of the prostate under treatment [1]. This is especially recommended for surgeons at their initial learning curves to measure the prostate size which provides an insight of anticipated difficulty especially in huge prostates. Oral anticoagulant therapy and/or platelet aggregation inhibitors would be stopped pre-operatively according to the patient's medical condition or regional medical guidelines, though it has been reported that these agents can be continued peri-operatively without excessive increase in transfusion rate and clot retention [16, 23].

2.2. Operative description of bipolar endoscopic enucleation of prostate

Our technique and experience of bipolar endoscopic enucleation of prostate has previously been reported [12]. The patient is put on general or spinal anesthesia with Lloyd-Davis position or lithotomy position. The operation is performed with continuous normal saline irrigation, 60–70 cm above the patient level. Cystoscopic examination of the lower urinary tract is performed to rule out any bladder malignancy or calculus. The ureteric orifice, bladder neck and the verumontanum are identified as the important landmark of bipolar endoscopic enucleation of the prostate.

Enucleation of the adenoma started from just proximal to the verumontanum at 5 and 7 o'clock. It aims to cleave the plane between the adenoma to the surgical capsule just proximal to the external urinary sphincter. The beak of the resectoscope could directly enter this plane through blunt dissection or an incision could be made over the urethral mucosa to the surgical capsule to start the enucleation but it may result in more bleeding and obscure the vision [18, 19]. This landmark is easily identifiable and the thickness of tissue that required to be cut is the thinnest. The surgeon should be able to visualize the whitish smooth surgical capsule of the prostate soon after opening up the urethral mucosa here. For bilobar BPE patient, enucleation is started just proximal to the verumontanum (**Figure 1**). Then, the plane between

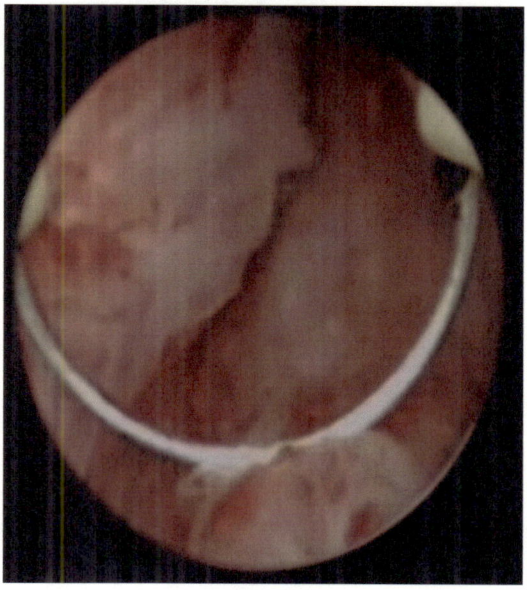

Figure 1. Incision of the urethral mucosa just proximal to verumontanum in case of enucleating bilobar enlarged prostate.

the adenoma and the capsule is developed by the beak of the resectoscope or by the bipolar electrode (**Figure 2**), depending on the preference of the surgeon and the available electrode. The distal mid lobe is dissected in retrograde fashion to the bladder neck. The blood vessels are coagulated by the bipolar electrode and the adhesive fibers are cut to open up the plane. The procedure is continued till the circular fiber of the bladder neck is identified (**Figure 3**). The bladder mucosa is incised to enter the bladder at 5 or 7 o'clock. Caution should be taken to dissect the posterior mid gland from the surgical capsule along the contour of the prostate posterior surface, so as to avoid perforation of the prostatic capsule and undermining the bladder neck at 6 o'clock.

The plane is further developed laterally with the suppling vessels coagulated. Both lateral lobes are enucleated laterally (**Figure 4**) to reach the 11 o'clock and 1 o'clock of the anterior fibromuscular stroma, where the adenoma is usually adhered more densely than the other region [17]. The attachment at 12 o'clock allows the adenoma be resected in the prostatic fossa rather than free floating inside the bladder.

Some urologists prefer to have enucleation of the prostate by starting from 5 or 7 o' clock proximal to the verumontanum and then bluntly dissected the adenoma laterally. The bladder was entered at 11 and 1 o'clock of the bladder neck to avoid entering the bladder over the trigone area. The anterior fibromuscular stroma at 12 o'clock was joined through the bilateral dissection plane and the adenoma was left attached to the bladder neck to facilitate adenoma resection.

After majority of the adenoma is devascularized, the adenoma is resected from the bladder neck by the loop electrode in an almost bloodless manner (**Figure 5**). The prostate chips are removed by Ellik's evacuator. As in usual bipolar transurethral resection of the prostate, gas

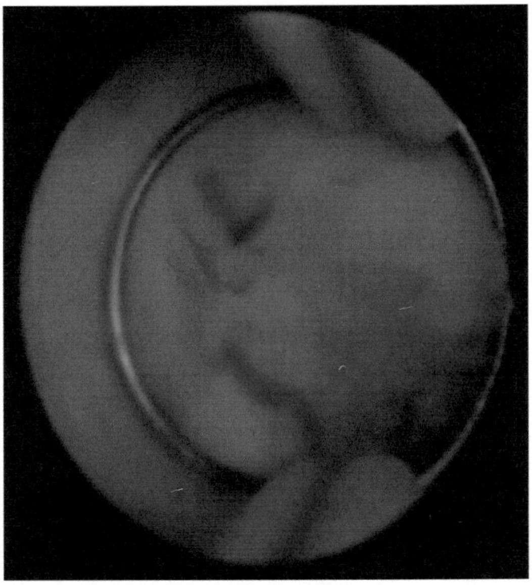

Figure 2. Development of the enucleation plane by using the beak and the bipolar electrode. The feeding vessels to the adenoma were coagulated.

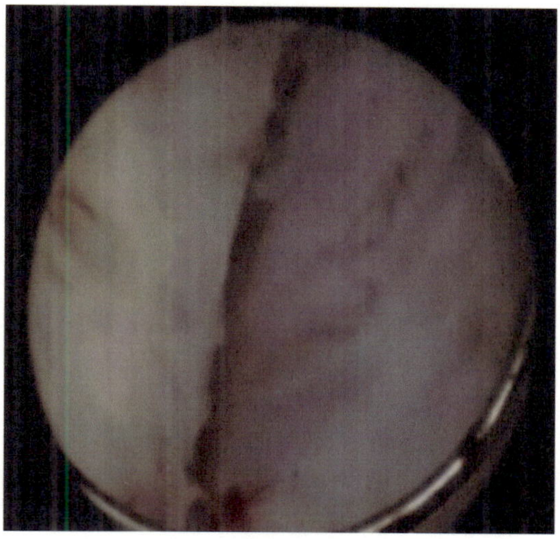

Figure 3. The enucleation process is continued till the circular muscle fiber of the bladder is noted.

will be accumulated inside the bladder and the intravesical pressure has been measured to be around 25 mmHg [17]. The increased intravesical pressure may obscure some venous bleeding. Careful hemostasis should be obtained after drainage of thee intravesical gas.

2.3. Tips and tricks of the technique of bipolar endoscopic enucleation of prostate

There are different kinds of bipolar transurethral systems reported in literature such as Gyrus PlasmaKinetic (PK) system, Olympus system through SurgMaster™ USE 40 generator

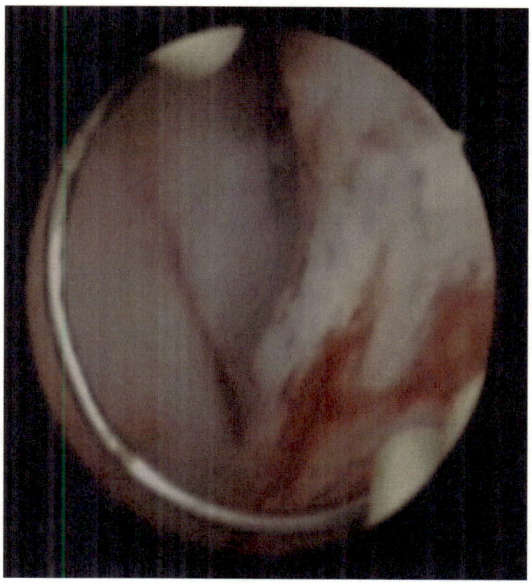

Figure 4. Enucleation of the lateral lobe of the adenoma.

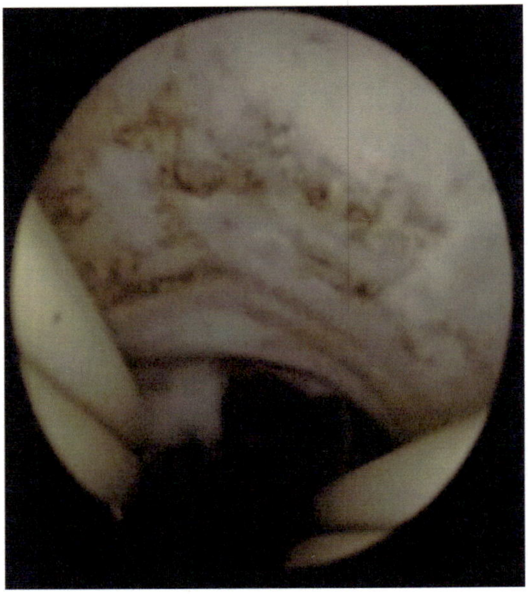

Figure 5. Resection of the devascularized adenoma from 6 o'clock from the bladder neck with the scope oriented upwards.

(Olympus Tokyo Japan) and Scanmed Plasmakinetic System (Scanmed, Zhuhai, China) [3, 7–19, 22]. However, it has been shown in that in Quasi-bipolar system which the electrical current is returned to the generator through the outer sheath of the bipolar resectoscope, the urethral stricture rate can be higher if the procedure is prolonged in larger prostate size >70 gm resection [24]. It is postulated that the return current over the out sheath may damage the bulbous urethra and causes an higher incidence of urethral stricture. However, this finding was reported in a single centre's experience [24] and was not observed in other groups' results using similar instruments [10, 19]. There will be some difference in design of the beak of the resectoscope and the strength of the electrode in different bipolar systems. The surgeon should be familarized with their instrument before deciding to use the beak or the electrode for enucleation.

Button electrode has been developed in both Gyrus PK and Olympus system. The button electrode has larger contact surface area and allows easier contact coagulation and vaporization. Button electrode has been used in bipolar endoscopic enucleation of the prostate [14, 15, 23] and it has been shown to provide better hemostasis especially for patients on anti-coagulation therapy [23]. The learning curve is also proposed to be shorter than the conventional bipolar endoscopic enucleation of prostate by using loop electrode [15]. However, these button electrodes are designed as single use items. Extra instruments such as loop electrode or morcellator are required for prostate adenoma resection on top of the use of button electrode. The Japanese group also reported the use of loop electrode with a specially designed spatula for blunt enucleation [13], though it is not readily available in other parts of the world.

In case of gross trilobar enlargement with prominent median lobe, 3-lobe technique can be considered [11, 18]. Incision is made at 5 and 7 o'clock of from the bladder neck to the verumontanum. The median lobe is enucleated and removed first. The procedure is continued with further enucleation of the lateral lobes through the same plane. The continuous normal saline irrigation is improved with the median lobe removed first.

A Chinese group described another enucleation technique to overcome the problem of enucleation of the prostate over the more densely adhered anterior fibromuscular stroma at 12 o'clock [17]. That region was firstly resected by bipolar transurethral resection of prostate down to the surgical capsule. The enucleation of the prostate is then started from verumontanum and then directed laterally to the 10 and 2 o'clock position. The adenoma is left attached to the bladder neck at 6 o'clock to avoid adenoma dislodgement into the bladder.

Despite adequate devascularization of the adenoma after enucleation, resection of the large adenoma with loop electrode can be difficult due to its size and disorientation, especially at the early learning curve. Our group resects the adneoma from 6 o'clock from the bladder neck with the scope oriented upwards, so that the resection of adenoma directed at 12 o'clock will not damage the surgical capsule [12]. Prof Liu utilized both forward and backward movement of the working element to resect the devascularized adenoma, in order to reduce the operative time [11]. Besides using the loop electrode for adenoma resection, morcellator is also used in some centers to reduce the adenoma resection time [13, 25], though caution should be taken to avoid bladder injury by the morcellator.

Although bipolar transurethral system allows the procedure to be safely performed in a longer period of time, it has been a concern if there is over-absorption of normal saline during the enucleation procedure especially with potential capsular perforation. Ran and his colleagues have compared the irrigation fluid absorption volume with bipolar enucleation and bipolar resection technique using 1% ethanol containing saline solution. It is found that there would be around 900 ml fluid absorbed for bipolar endoscopic enucleation with around 70 gm prostate [26] and it was not different from bipolar transurethral resection of the prostate with similar size. Especially in patients with underlying cardiovascular conditions, it is advisable to give frusemide intra-operatively to reduce the chance of fluid overload [11].

3. Surgical outcome of bipolar endoscopic enucleation of prostate

3.1. Functional outcome

Current literature demonstrated bipolar endoscopic enucleation of prostate could achieve functional outcome comparable to open prostatectomy. Data drawn from bipolar endoscopic enucleation of prostate arm of 5 randomized control trials for prostate size >80 ml [3, 17] showed that bipolar endoscopic enucleation of prostate reduced lower urinary tract symptoms by 83% (76–86%, with reduction of IPSS point 17.6–22.1), improved quality of life (QOL) score by 70% (50–82%), increased mean maximum urine flow (Qmax) by 331% (152–535%, +9.6–21.4 ml/s), and reduced post voiding residual volume (PVR) by 86% (68–93%). Efficacy was maintained for up to 6 years [5].

For perioperative outcomes, it was reported that the resected specimen's weight could reach a mean of 80.4% of the preoperative prostate size. Average operative time was 109 min [3, 5, 6, 17] with a mean prostate size of 111 cc, and this was likely achieved by surgeons that have passed the learning curve. With the use of morcellator operative time could be further shortened, as demonstrated in one randomized control trial [4] the operative time was 87 mins with a mean prostate size of 123 cc.

The randomized controlled trials reported the catheterization time to be 2.3 days, and the average length of stay was 4.2 days. Re-catheterization due to retention ranged from 0 to 4.3%.

3.2. Complications

For early complications, transient stress urinary incontinence was reported ranging from 0 to 8.75%. One randomized controlled trial reported early storage urinary symptoms to be 2.1% [17]. Mean hemoglobin drop of 1.16 g/dL with blood transfusion rate ranging from 0 to 6.4%. UTI was reported ranging 3.6–7%. There was a small chance of clot retention 0–1.1%.

For late complications, bladder neck contracture/stenosis was reported to be 0–2.4%, urethral stricture was reported as 2.1–3.75%. There was no permanent incontinence reported in this 5 RCT, and no reoperation for regeneration of adenoma was reported.

3.3. Learning curve

Xiong et al. evaluated the learning curve of the initial 100 cases of 2 surgeons. It was reported that the surgeons required 30 operations until a few conversions to conventional bipolar TURP occurred [19]. It also noted that 50 operations were required to achieved a stable surgical efficiency, as measured by mL/minute of tissue being enucleated and resected. This was echoed by another Japanese single surgeon cohort [13], which showed the efficiency improved markedly when the surgeon experience exceeded the initial 50 cases. With the presence of mentor, 40 cases was required to reach plateau in terms of operation or enucleation efficiency in g/min, as shown in one retrospective study [27].

Barriers during the learning curve focused on properly identifying and handling the right plane in the absence of mentorship. The anatomic landmarks that prompt the surgeon to identify the surgical plane mainly include capsule transverse fibers or fiber strands, capsule vessel reticula, capsule prostate calculi [19].

The advantage of bipolar endoscopic enucleation of prostate during the learning curve is that it can be converted to conventional bipolar transurethral resection of prostate, using the same set of instrument with no harm to patients. Though Tracey et al. reported a higher rate of capsular perforation or undermining of the bladder neck in the initial learning curve in up to 8% [28].

4. Comparison with other surgical modality for BPH

4.1. Open prostatectomy

Bipolar endoscopic enucleation of prostate was most frequently compared with open prostatectomy in the current available literature as open prostatectomy is still be regarded as the gold standard surgical procedure for large benign prostate enlargement. Four randomized control trials were available [3–6]. All these studies showed the functional outcome were similar but bipolar endoscopic enucleation of the prostate improved perioperative parameters in terms of less hemoglobin drop, less transfusion, shorter catheterization time and shorter length of stay. The wound complications related to open surgery were avoided including wound dehiscence, wound infection and paralytic ileus reported [5]. There was no significant difference in other mid and long term complications in terms of bladder neck stenosis, urethral stricture. In the European Association of Urology guideline 2018, endoscopic enucleation (including bipolar energy) was rated as first recommended choice for treating substantially enlarged prostate ≥80 gm, same as open prostatectomy (previous gold standard), with a more favorable peri-operative safety profile [1].

4.2. Bipolar transurethral resection of prostate

Two randomized control trials [4, 17] compared bipolar TURP with bipolar endoscopic enucleation of prostate. The surgical efficacy was higher for bipolar endoscopic enucleation of prostate with more resected weight as compare to bipolar TURP. At 12 month follow-up, persistent significant difference in Qmax, IPSS and QOL was shown in one randomized controlled trial [17] but not for another one [4]. Significantly higher perioperative complications in terms of clot retention, dysuria, re-catheterization, blood transfusion, and reoperation for bipolar TURP were reported in one randomized controlled study [17].

4.3. Photoselective vaporization of prostate (PVP)

One prospective cohort compared PVP (160 W LBO green laser system) with bipolar endoscopic enucleation of prostate. It demonstrated that significant improvement of IPSS, QOL, Qmax, PVR and PSA changes in favor of bipolar endoscopic enucleation of prostate in 12 months (mean prostate size 88.3 ml) [21]. There was no difference in terms of perioperative complications and no transfusion was required in both group of patient.

4.4. Holmium laser enucleation of prostate (HoLEP)

One small randomized control trial (n = 40) compared HoLEP and bipolar endoscopic enucleation of prostate in medium sized prostate (mean 51 cc) [10]. The author commented bipolar endoscopic enucleation of prostate had more pronounced postoperative irrigation requirement because of reduced visibility and a greater propensity for bleeding as compared with HoLEP. Longer operative time was noted for bipolar endoscopic enucleation of prostate. However, it was still the early infancy of the development in bipolar endoscopic enucleation of prostate on the study period. The result was likely due to the comparison of initial development of bipolar endoscopic enucleation of prostate to more well established HoLEP technique in the study period. Other perioperative parameters/complications are similar without significant difference between both groups.

4.5. Thulium laser enucleation of prostate (ThuLEP)

A randomized control trial [20] compared ThuLEP with bipolar endoscopic enucleation of prostate in medium sized prostate (mean 67.1 cc). ThuLEP provided less risk of hemorrhage and shorter catheter time, although the differences may be of little clinical relevance. No statistical differences in complications between the two groups. Assessment at 12-month follow-up showed no difference in urinary parameters between the two groups.

5. Conclusion

Bipolar endoscopic enucleation of prostate provides an excellent minimally invasive modality for surgical treatment of large BPE especially for those ≥80 gm. It allowed better functional outcome than transurethral resection and stepwise adenoma devascularization with minimally invasive technique. The instruments were familiar to most urologists and were available in most modernly equipped urology centers. In addition, it allows easy and quick conversion to traditional transurethral resection. The authors believe endoscopic enucleation of the prostate including bipolar energy has replaced open prostatectomy as the standard of care in the surgical management of large BPE.

Conflict of interest

There is no conflict of interest to be declared by the authors.

Author details

Wai Hee Steve Chan[1]*, Chi Fai Kan[2] and Churk Fai Trevor Li[2]

*Address all correspondence to: stevewh@gmail.com

1 Hong Kong Sanatorium and Hospital, Hong Kong SAR, China

2 Queen Elizabeth Hosptial, Hong Kong SAR, China

References

[1] Gravas S, Cornu JN, Drake MJ, et al. Non-neurogenic male lower urinary tract symptoms (LUTS), incl. Benign prostatic obstruction (BPO). EAU guidelines. Edn. Presented at the EAU Annual Congress Copenhagen; 2018. ISBN 978-94-92671-01-1

[2] Mayer EK, Kroeze SGC, Chopra S, Bottle A, Patel A. Examining the 'gold standard': A comparative critical analysis of three decades of monopolar transurethral resection of the prostate (TURP) outcome. BJU International. 2012 Dec;**110**(11):1595-1601. DOI: 10.1111/j.1464-410X.2012.11119.x.a

[3] Rao JM, Yang JR, Ren YX, He J, Ding P, Yang JH. Plasmakinetic enucleation of the prostate versus transvesical open prostatectomy for benign prostatic hyperplasia >80 mL: 12-month follow-up results of a randomized clinical trial. Urology. 2013;**82**:176

[4] Geavlete B, Bulai C, Ene C, Checherita I, Geavlete P. Bipolar vaporization, resection, and Enucleation versus open prostatectomy: Optimal treatment alternatives in large prostate cases? Journal of Endourology. 2015;**29**(3):323-331. http://doi.org/10.1089/end.2014.0493

[5] Chen S, Zhu L, Cai J, Zheng Z, Ge R, Wu M, et al. Plasmakinetic enucleation of the prostate compared with open prostatectomy for prostates larger than 100 grams: A randomized noninferiority controlled trial with long-term results at 6 years. European Urology. 2014;**66**(2):284-291. http://doi.org/10.1016/j.eururo.2014.01.010

[6] Ou R, Deng X, Yang W, Wei X, Chen H, Xie K. Transurethral enucleation and resection of the prostate vs transvesical prostatectomy for prostate volumes >80 mL: A prospective randomized study. BJU International. 2013;**112**(2):239-245. http://doi.org/10.1111/bju.12181

[7] Hiraoka Y. A new method of prostatectomy, transurethral detachment and resection of benign prostatic hyperplasia. Nihon Ika Daiqaku Zasshi. 1983 Dec;**50**(6):896-898

[8] Lin Y, Wu X, Xu A, Ren R, et al. Transurethral enucleation of the prostate versus transvesical open prostatectomy for large benign prostatic hyperplasia: A systematic review and meta-analysis of randomized controlled trials. World Journal of Urology. 2016;**34**: 1207-1219. DOI: 10.1007/s00345-015-1735-9

[9] Fraundorfer MR, Gilling PJ. Holmium:YAG laser enucleation of the prostate combined with mechanical morcellation: Preliminary results. European Urology; **33**(1):69-72

[10] Neill MG, Gilling PJ, Kennett KM, Framptom CM, Westenberg AM, Fraundorfer MR, Wilson LC. Randomized trial comparing holmium laser enucleation of prostate with plasmakinetic enucleation of prostate for treatment of benign prostatic hyperplasia. Urology. 2006;**68**(5):1020-1024. DOI: 10.1016/j.urology.2006.06.021

[11] Liu C, Zheng S, Li H, Xu K. Transurethral enucleation and resection of prostate in patients with benign prostatic hyperplasia by plasma kinetics. Journal of Urology. 2010;**184**:2440-2445. DOI: 10.106/j.juro.2010.08.037

[12] Kan CF, Tsu HL, Chiu Y, To HC, Sze B, Chan SWH. A prospective study comparing bipolar endoscopic enucleation of prostate with bipolar transurethral resection in saline for management of symptomatic benign prostatic enlargement larger than 70g in a matched cohort. International Urology and Nephrology. 2014;**46**:51-517. DOI: 10.1007/s11255-013-0546-4

[13] Hirasawa Y, Kato Y, Fujita. Transurethral enucleation with bipolar for benign prostatic hyperplasia: 2-year outcomes and the learning curve of a single surgeon's experience of 603 consecutive patients. Journal of Endourology. 2017;**31**(7):679-685. DOI: 10.1089/end.2017.0092

[14] Geavlete B, Stanescu F, Lacoboaie C, Geavlete P. Bipolar plasma enucleation of the prostate vs open prostatectomy in large benign prostatic hyperplasia cases – A medium term, prospective, randomized comparison. BJU International. 2013;**111**:793-803. DOI: 10.1111/j.1464-410X.2012.11730.x

[15] Abou-Taleb A, El-Shaer W, Kandeel W, Gharib T, Elshaer A. Bipolar plamakinetic enucleoresection of the prostate: Our experience with 245 patients for 3 years of follow-up. Journal of Endourology. 2017;**31**(3):300-306. DOI: 10.1089/end.2016.0746

[16] El-Shaer W, Abou-Taleb A, Kandeel W. Transurethral bipolar plasmakinetic vapo-enucleation of the prostate: Is it safe for patients on chronic oral anticoagulants and/or platelet

aggregation inhibitors? Arab Journal of Urology. 2017;**15**:347-354. https://doi.org/10.1016/j.aju.2017.09.005

[17] Li K, Wang D, Hu C, et al. A novel modification of transurethral enucleation and resection of the prostate in patients with prostate glands larger than 80 ml: Surgical procedures and clinical outcomes. Urology. 2018;**113**:153-159. http://doi.org/10.1016/j.urology.2017.11.036

[18] Cho CL, Leung CLH, Chan WKW, Chu RWH, Law IC. Early post-operative outcome of bipolar transurethral enucleation and resection of the prostate. Hong Kong Medical Journal. 2015;**21**(6):528-535

[19] Xiong W, Sun M, Ran Q, Chen F, Du Y, Dou K. Learning curve for bipolar transurethral enucleation and resection of the prostate in saline for symptomatic benign prostatic hyperplasia: Experience in the first 100 consecutive patients. Urologia Internationalis. 2013;**90**:68-74. DOI: 10.1159/000343235

[20] Feng L, Zhang D, Tian Y, Song J. Thulium laser Enucleation versus Plasmakinetic Enucleation of the prostate: A randomized trial of a single center. Journal of Endourology. 2016;**30**(6):665-670. http://doi.org/10.1089/end.2015.0867

[21] Mu XN, Wang SJ, Chen J, Jin XB, Huang ZX, Zhang LY. Bipolar Transurethral Enucleation of Prostate Versus Photoselective Vaporization for Symptomatic Benign Prostatic Hyperplasia (>70 Ml); 2017. pp. 608-612. http://doi.org/10.4103/1008-682X.178484

[22] Nicolle L, Bradley S, Colgan R, Rice JC, Schaeffer A, Hooton T. Clinical Infectious Diseases. 2005;**40**(5):643-654

[23] Giolianelli R, Gentile B, Albanesi L, Tariciotti P, Mirabile G. Urology. 2015;**86**(2):407-414. http://dx.dot.org/10.1016/j.urology.2015.03.045

[24] Komura K, Inamoto T, Takai T, et al. Incidence of urethral stricture after bipolar transurethral resection of the prostate using TURis: Results from a randomized trial. BJU International. 2015 Apr;**115**(4):644-652. DOI: 10.1111/bju.12831

[25] Naspro R, Sancha FG, Manica M, et al. From "gold standard" resection to reproducible "future standard" endoscopic enucleation of the prostate: What we know about anatomical enucleation. Minerva Urologica e Nefrologica. 2016 Oct;**69**(5):446-458. DOI: 10.23736/S0393-2249.17.02834-X

[26] Ran L, He W, Zhu X, Zhou Q, Goui X. Comparison of fluid absorption between transurethral enucleation and transurethral resection for benign prostate hyperplasia. Urologia Internationalis. 2013;**91**:26-30. DOI: 10.1159/000348793

[27] Feng L, Song J, Zhang D, Tian Y. Evaluation of the learning curve for transurethral plasmakinetic enucleation and resection of prostate using a mentor-based approach. International Brazilian Journal of Urology. 2017;**43**(2):245-255. http://doi.org/10.1590/S1677-5538.IBJU.2016.0237

[28] Tracey JM, Warner JN. Transurethral bipolar Enucleation of the prostate is an effective treatment option for men with urinary retention. Urology. 2016;**87**:166-171. http://doi.org/10.1016/j.urology.2015.10.011

Section 5

Simple Prostatectomy Technique - Laparoscopic Simple Prostatectomy

Chapter 5

Laparoscopic Simple Prostatectomy

Yusuf Ilker Comez

Additional information is available at the end of the chapter

http://dx.doi.org/10.5772/intechopen.79549

Abstract

Benign prostatic hyperplasia (BPH) is the most common benign tumor and cause of urinary retention in middle-aged male patients. Transurethral resection of the prostate (TURP) is the gold standard surgical treatment for benign prostatic obstruction. Although widely performed, TURP is associated with significant morbidity. Open prostatectomy is performed in larger glands, which are more than 80 grams, with higher morbidity. Advances in technology, such as holmium laser enucleation of the prostate (HoLEP) and KTP laser vaporization, are other options that are widely used despite their limitations. Laparoscopic simple prostatectomy (LSP) is a minimally invasive treatment option with equivalent functional outcomes and is useful in larger prostatic adenomas, with low morbidity in experienced hands.

Keywords: prostatectomy, adenomectomy, prostatic adenoma, benign prostatic hyperplasia, laparoscopy, minimally invasive, simple prostatectomy

1. Introduction

Benign prostatic hyperplasia (BPH) is the most common benign pathology and cause of urinary retention in middle-aged male patients, and its incidence increases with age.

The International Prostate Symptom Score (IPSS) questionnaire is often used to assess patients of BPH [1]. The treatment depends on the severity of the disease. Conservative approach with watchful waiting and the use of systemic drugs that relaxes the smooth muscles of the prostate and bladder neck, resulting in the decrease in the prostate mass volume, may be preferred in the mild cases. When planning surgery, prostate volume and weight as well as the patients' expectations and associated comorbidities should be taken into account.

In patients with failure or inability to tolerate medical treatment, with urinary retention, renal failure secondary to BPH, urinary infections, bladder calculi, or hematuria, surgical intervention should be preferred [2–5].

Transurethral prostate resection (TURP), simple prostatectomy, and transurethral incision of the prostate (TUIP) have been the main surgical treatment options for benign prostate hyperplasia (BPH) for decades. Although TURP is accepted as the gold standard surgical treatment for benign prostatic obstruction and is widely used in all over the world, it has several limitations such as being insufficient in treating large prostates, risk of perioperative bleeding, postoperative transurethral resection (TUR) syndrome, urethral strictures, and at the same time the risk of reoperation requirement [6].

EAU and AUA guidelines recommend open prostatectomy (OP) for the surgical treatment of patients with prostate volumes larger than 80 ml [7, 8]. The advantages of this technique are lower reoperation rates and better clinical outcomes with more patient satisfaction [9]. However, it has also been associated with the need for perioperative transfusion, prolonged hospital stay, higher reoperation rate, urinary infections, and a large abdominal scar effecting the cosmesis [10–12]. Other rare adverse events as clot retention, contraction in the bladder neck, wound infection, and myocardial infarction may also be encountered [13]. Holmium laser enucleation of the prostate (HoLEP) is used in larger adenomas as an alternative to OP with the advantages such as shorter catheterization and hospital stay. However, the technique is not widely used because of the demanding learning curve, complications, and the need for special equipment [6].

The other laser treatment option as an alternative to OP is the GreenLight® KTP laser vaporization that promised better outcomes for large prostate adenomas with successful results [14]. By this technique surgeons achieved shorter catheterization time and hospital stay with perfect hemostasis [14]. However, the absence of definitive pathological result and lack of long-term results were the obstacles for the widespread use of the technique.

With advancements in the technology, minimal invasive methods such as enucleation of the prostate with holmium laser or laparoscopic simple prostatectomy (LSP) began to show off on stage.

LSP is recently accepted as an alternative to open surgery in patients with large prostate glands. However, it is accepted that learning curve of this technique is steep and time-consuming in order to reach to comparable results to OP [15].

In this chapter the benefits, conflicts, and surgical technique of laparoscopic simple prostatectomy are described with the review of the literature.

2. The surgical technique for simple laparoscopic prostatectomy

The surgical procedures may be performed either in an extraperitoneal or transperitoneal fashion [16–18].

Adenomectomy can be performed transvesically or by retropubic transcapsular (Millin) technique [19].

2.1. Port placement

The laparoscopic simple prostatectomy begins with placement of the trocars either transperitoneally or extraperitoneally [19, 20].

Intubation and nasogastric decompression are applied at supine position. The bladder emptying is performed after insertion of 22-F Foley catheter. Afterward, the spread of the legs to 30° at Trendelenburg position is performed. Both arms are fixed adjacent to the body (**Figure 1A**).

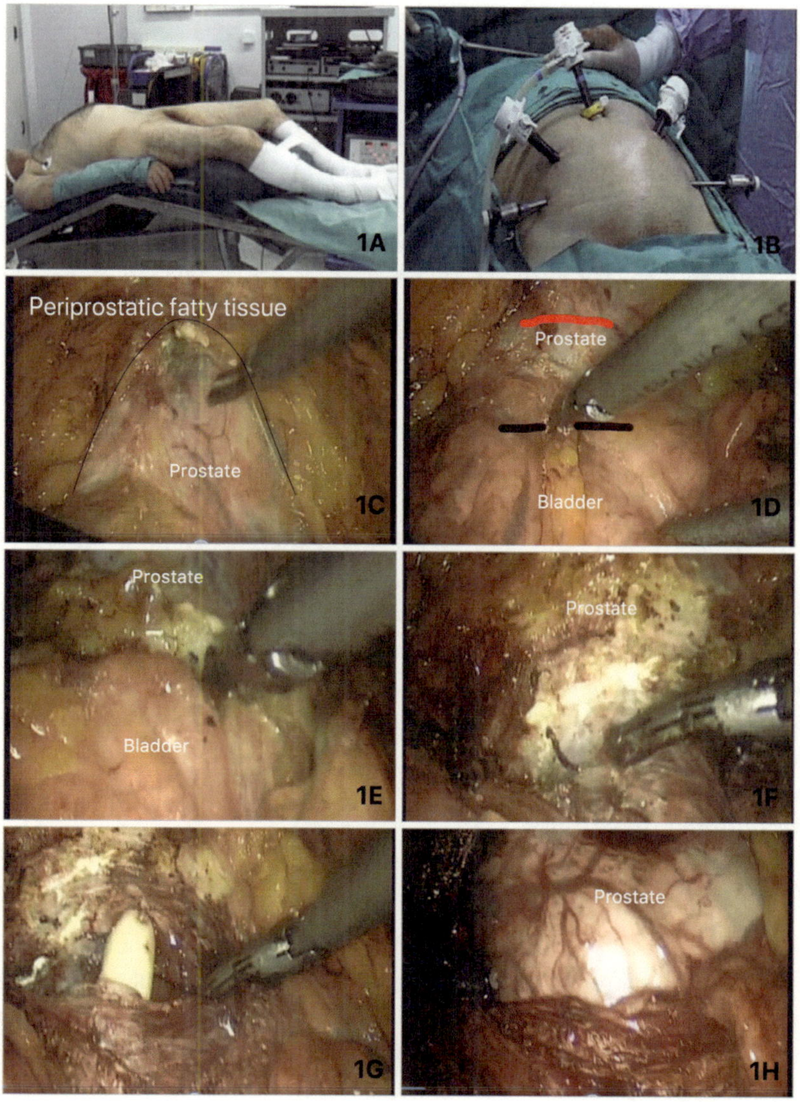

Figure 1. (A) The position of the patient for LSP; (B) the port placement for LSP; (C) the defatting the tissue over the prostate capsule; (D) black line shows the incision 1-cm proximal to the prostatovesical junction in transvesical approach; the red line depicts the ventral incision over prostate in retropubic transvesical Millin technique; (E) dissection of the detrussor with harmonic scissors; (F) widening the incision to see both orifices and prostate; (G) intravesical part of the Foley catheter is seen; and (H) the intravesical portion of the prostate can easily be pulled out of the fossa.

2.1.1. The extraperitoneal approach

The extraperitoneal approach involves making a 30-mm infraumbilical incision and dissecting down to the anterior rectus fascia. This fascia is incised 30 mm transversely, and after demonstrating the linea alba and rectus muscles, the bellies of the rectus are separated bluntly in the midline. Finger dissection is carried out between the rectus muscle and the peritoneum to form the preperitoneal space, taking care to avoid incidental peritonotomy by applying anterior pressure inferiorly when the posterior rectus fascia disappears below the arcuate line. Linea alba is incised adjacent to symphysis pubis inferiorly. A 12-mm balloon dissector with 10-mm visual optical channel is placed to the preperitoneal space superior to the bladder and the prostate. Anterior rectus fascia defect, near to the port, is closed. Subcutaneous and cutaneous sutures are performed with No.1 silk sutures to avoid gas leakage. The balloon is slowly inflated under direct visualization in the retroperitoneum. In the correct plane, the inferior epigastric vessels are visible ventrally helping to avoid incidental vascular damage. The balloon is deinflated, the 10-mm trocar and a 0-degree optical lens are inserted, and the space is inflated with 10–15 mmHg of CO_2. Four additional trocars are inserted under direct visualization. Two 10-mm trocars are placed lateral to the rectus muscle over the line between anterior superior iliac spine and the umbilicus, and two 5-mm trocars are placed 2 cm medial to the anterior superior iliac spines (**Figure 1B**).

2.1.2. The transperitoneal approach

The transperitoneal approach is performed with the Trendelenburg position as described previously. A 2-mm incision below the umbilicus is performed. After reaching the rectus fascia, Veress needle is inserted in the peritoneum carefully. After forming pneumoperitoneum, a 10-mm port is replaced with 2-cm port inferior to the umbilicus in the midline between the rectus muscles. The other ports are replaced under direct visualization similar to the retroperitoneal approach. As we reach to the bladder, the peritoneum is incised ventrally to the bladder. By the caudal dissection via peritoneal incision, Retzius space is reached. The next steps of the surgery are similar either extraperitoneal or transperitoneal. As we reach the Retzius space, defatting the tissue over the prostate for better visualization of the prostate and bladder neck is provided (**Figure 1C**).

2.2. The techniques of dissection

2.2.1. The transvesical dissection technique

The bladder is filled with 200 cc saline. Therefore, careful manipulation of the bladder helps to identify prostatic lobes from the softer bladder wall. If transvesical approach is chosen, a transverse incision is done 2 cm proximally to the prostatovesical junction with harmonic scissors (**Figure 1D**). After transverse cystostomy, one may widen the incision laterally (**Figure 1F**), until the large adenoma can be seen clearly (**Figure 1H**). A grasper can also be used for anterior elevation of the median lobe to see the bladder lumen and orifices clearly (**Figure 2A**). Afterward, the Foley catheter is pulled out, and metal bugi is replaced to lift the prostate superiorly. Adequate vision allows the dissection of the adenoma through a transverse incision distal to the trigone (**Figure 2B** and **C**). The bladder neck is well perfused, and the use of harmonic scissors may be useful to prevent bleeding. Suction and posterior traction by the assistant are

http://dx.doi.org/10.5772/intechopen.79549

mandatory. The subcapsular plane can be identified by leaving prostatic capsule posteriorly and elevating the adenoma out of the fossa. In the subcapsular plane, the aspirator is used for blunt dissection, while sharp dissections are made with harmonic scissor (**Figure 2D**). Prostatic tissue is liberated from 6-o'clock to 12-o'clock position in both sides (**Figure 2E** and **F**). In this stage of surgery, the use of suction and harmonic scissors may prevent vision difficulty due to bleeding (**Figure 2G** and **H**). Minor bleedings may be ignored. The pneumoperitoneum may

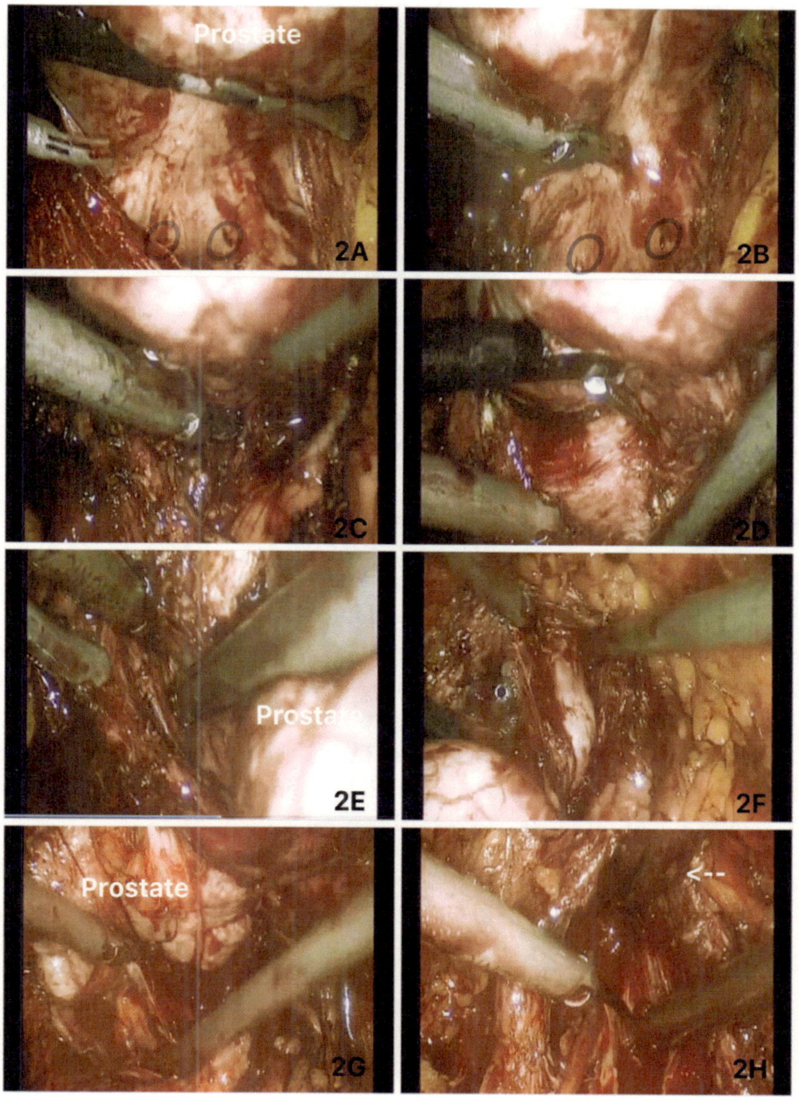

Figure 2. (A) a grasper can also be used for anterior elevation of the median lobe to see the bladder lumen and orifices clearly. Both orifices are shown in a black circle; (B) the harmonic dissection of the adenoma through a transverse incision distal to the trigone to enter the subcapsular space; (C) releasing the adenoma; (E) dissection to separate left side of the adenoma from the capsule. A grasper helps for traction while blunt and sharp dissections are held with harmonic scissors; (F) dissection of the anterior part of the right lobe; and (G and H) the releasing of the last posterior adhesions with the help of the superior adenoma lifting.

facilitate better vision (**Figure 3A**). In extremely large prostates, it may be required to resect the median lobe priorly. The anterior plane is then approached and followed caudally. The extent of the resection begins proximally from the bladder neck, distally to the verumontanum. Care must be given not to injure the urethra and the sphincter (**Figure 3B**). The adenoma is enucleated and placed into a specimen bag (**Figure 3C**). If the adenoma is extremely large, it may be cut into small pieces by endoscissors and put in the specimen bag to secure.

Once the adenoma is enucleated, the pneumoperitoneum provides better visualization of arterial capsular bleeders that can be controlled with harmonic scissors. If bladder neck bleedings originate from the intravesical pedicle, ligation with V-loc hemostatic sutures or placement of M-knots with a 3-0 Vicryl can be used. Trigonization is described as plication of the bladder neck over the posterior capsule and performed in an interrupted fashion with 2-0 monocryl sutures (**Figure 3D** and **E**). The aim of this technique is to ensure the passage of the Foley catheter from the urethra into the bladder. Urethrovesical anastomosis has been proposed to ensure apposition of the bladder neck to urethral mucosa while helping the hemostasis and allegedly decreasing bladder neck contracture rates [21].

At the end of the hemostasis and trigonization, 22-F Foley catheter is replaced to the bladder, and cystostomy is closed with 2-0 Vicryl with interrupted sutures (van Velthoven technique) (**Figure 3F** and **G**) [22]. After closing the cystectomy, the balloon is filled with 30-ml saline, and urinary leakage is controlled by filling the bladder (**Figure 3H**). A Jackson Pratt drain is replaced to the Retzius space. Specimen is taken out from the port below the umbilicus.

2.2.2. Laparoscopic transcapsular (Millin) technique

The retropubic approach can be done utilizing several incisions. Transverse anterior prostatic, longitudinal anterior prostatic incisions and longitudinal prostatovesical and transverse incision just proximal to the prostatovesical junction are some of the choices. Sotelo et al. described their technique as they use the transverse incision adjacent to the prostatovesical junction. This technique avoids bleeding of the venous plexus. The other recommendation of Sotelo et al. is resection of the adenoma as separate lobes for improved visualization [21]. The use of suprapubic hand port is another modified technique. The hand port usage improves the speed of resection and provides hemostatic control [22].

The superiority of the transvesical technique over transcapsular (Millin) technique is identifying the intravesical median lob and allowing the dissection without injuring the orifices.

Regardless of the type of dissection chosen, the bladder irrigation for 24 h and urethral catheterization for 3–4 days are adequate postoperatively.

2.3. Complications

A complete cardiovascular workup should be performed during patient selection and surgical planning. Major complications are incontinence, bleeding, and cardiac complications. They account for much of the morbidity and mortality.

Patients should be screened for prostate cancer before undergoing surgery. The incidental prostate cancer rates may increase up to 10% of specimens in larger series [16, 23–30].

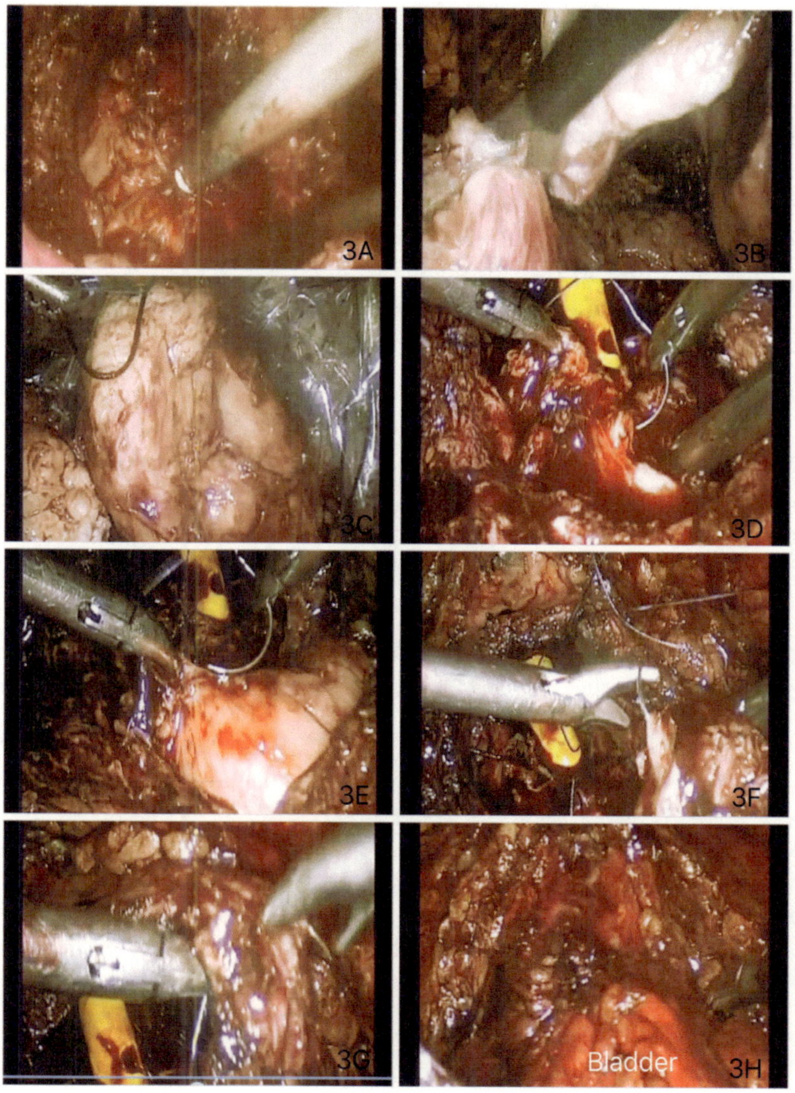

Figure 3. (A) The residual bleedings at the fossa are controlled by harmonic scissors; (B) the last adhesions are separated by endoscissors; (C) the adenoma is placed in the endobag; (D) the bleedings at the fossa are controlled with 3/0 Vicryl or V-loc hemostatic sutures; (E) trigonization is performed with plication of the bladder neck over the posterior capsule and facilitated in an interrupted fashion with 2-0 monocryl; (F and G) after 22-F Foley catheter is replaced to the bladder, cystostomy is closed with 2/0 Vicryl interrupted sutures; and (H) the bladder is finally filled with 200-ml saline in order to see if there is any leakage.

3. Discussion

Schuessler performed first laparoscopic radical prostatectomy in 1991 [31]. In 2002 Mariano et al. and in 2005 Sotelo et al. also performed laparoscopic simple prostatectomy for BPH [20, 21]. Mariano et al. reported first results of laparoscopic prostatectomy in 60 BPH patients with mean prostate weight of 144.50 ± 41.74 g. The mean operation time was 138.48 ± 23.38 min with blood loss of 330.98 ± 149.52 mL and without any postoperative urinary incontinence [20]. Sotelo and van Velthoven et al., with minor modifications with the surgical technique, reported similar successful results without postoperative complications [21, 22].

Although initial results are encouraging, and its benefits including less blood loss and shorter hospital stay are better than the open surgery, there are very limited studies in the literature comparing the results of LSP with open prostatectomy [23, 32–34]. Most studies report the results of the small case series of LSP with different surgical approaches such as extraperitoneal, transperitoneal, transcapsular, or finger-assisted approaches [19–22, 31, 35–37]. In the literature, the results of extraperitoneal or transperitoneal techniques are reported to be similar without any superiority to the other [16–18].

Hoepffner et al., in their study with the biggest series published, reported 100 patients' results with mean prostate weight of 97.1 ± 18.5 g, mean operation time 66.3 ± 12.3 min with blood loss of 250 ± 86.8 ml without the need of blood transfusion with mean hospital stay of 4.2 ± 1.3 days and mean catheterization time of 3.2 ± 1 days [38]. Oktay et al. reported the results of 16 LSP patients with the biggest prostate weight, 147 g (between 80 and 200 g), mean operation time 133 min (75–210 min), mean blood loss 134 ml (50–300 ml) requiring one transfusion, hospital stay 3.9 days (2–7 days), and catheterization duration of 6.3 (6–7) days [39].

Chlosta et al.., in their series of 66 patients, reported surgery time of 55 (45–85) minutes as the shortest surgery time and similar results for blood loss, hospital stay, and catheterization time [40].

There are four studies comparing the results of LSP with open prostatectomy. Three studies with small number of patients reported less blood loss [23, 32, 33], less hospitalization time [17, 18, 20], and less catheterization time [32–34]. One study with bigger number of patients, by McCullough et al., compared the results of 96 LSP patients with 184 open prostatectomy patients and found no statistically significant difference in blood loss (350 vs. 400 ml) and in prostate volume (111.3 vs. 117.2 g) between two techniques; however, statistically significant differences were found in terms of hospitalization time (6.3 vs. 7.7 days) ($p < 0.001$) and catheterization time (5.2 vs. 6.4 days) ($p < 0.001$) [34].

Porpiglia et al. reported statistically significant difference in blood loss between two techniques. Although the operation time, hospitalization, and catheterization time were longer in LSP than in the open prostatectomy, no significant differences are reported [23].

4. Conclusion

Simple prostatectomy although is still the treatment of choice in larger prostates and may be performed effectively via several techniques, newer technologies offer minimally invasive techniques for both patients and surgeons. If patients are able to reach or purchase, the outcomes may increasingly be better. It is obvious that LSP has as steep learning curve comparable to open prostatectomy but is a minimally invasive surgery and has satisfying results in larger prostates with low morbidity and hospital stay in the hand of experienced surgeons. Our goal is the final outcome of improved LUTS and decreasing residual volume while minimizing the cost and the complications.

Acknowledgements

I would like to express my special thanks to Prof. Dr. Hakan Vuruskan and Dr. Kadir Omur Gunseren for sharing their surgical photos.

Conflict of interest

No conflict of interest.

Author details

Yusuf Ilker Comez

Address all correspondence to: icomez@hotmail.com

Canakkale Government Hospital, Department of Urology, Canakkale, Turkey

References

[1] Barry MJ, Fowler FJ Jr, O'Leary MP, et al. The American Urological Association symptom index for benign prostatic hyperplasia. The Measurement Committee of the American Urological Association. Journal of Urology. 1992;**148**:1549-1557

[2] Sarma AV, Jacobson DJ, McGree ME, Roberts RO, Lieber MM, Jacobsen SJ. A population based study of incidence and treatment of benign prostatic hyperplasia among residents of Olmsted County, Minnesota: 1987 to 1997. The Journal of Urology. 2005;**173**:2048-2053

[3] McVary KT, Roehrborn CG, Avins AL, Barry MJ, Bruskewitz RC, Donnell RF, Foster HE Jr, Gonzalez CM, Kaplan SA, Penson DF, Ulchaker JC, Wei JT. Update on AUA guideline on the management of benign prostatic hyperplasia. The Journal of Urology. 2011;**185**:1793-1803

[4] de la Rosette JJ, Alivizatos G, Madersbacher S, Perachino M, Thomas D, Desgrandchamps F, de Wildt M, European Association of Urology. EAU guidelines on benign prostatic hyperplasia (BPH). European Urology. 2001;**40**:256-263. DOI: 10.1159/000049784

[5] Parsons JK, Wilt TJ, Wang PY, Barrett-Connor E, Bauer DC, Marshall LM, Osteoporotic Fractures in Men Research Group. Progression of lower urinary tract symptoms in older men: A community based study. The Journal of Urology. 2010;**183**:1915-1920

[6] Reich O, Gratzke C, Stief CG. Techniques and long-term results of surgical procedures for BPH. European Urology. 2006;**49**:970-978

[7] http://www.uroweb.org/index.php?structure_id=140#EAU_guidelines_online

[8] http://www.auanet.org/guidelines/

[9] Asimakopoulos AD, Mugnier C, Hoepffner J, Lopez L, Re D, Gaston R, Piechaud T Laparoscopic treatment of benign prostatic hyperplasia (BPH): Overview of the current techniques. BJU International. 2011;**107**:1168-1182. DOI: 10.1111/j.1464-410X.2011.10157.x

[10] Serretta V, Morgia G, Fondacaro L, Curto G, Lobianco A, Pirritano D, Melloni D, Orestano F, Motta M, Pavone-Macaluso M, Members of the Sicilian-Calabrian Society of Urology. Open prostatectomy for benign prostatic enlargement in southern Europe in the late 1990s: A contemporary series of 1800 interventions. Urology. 2002;**60**(4):623-627

[11] Gratzke C, Schlenker B, Seitz M, Karl A, Hermanek P, Lack N, Stief CG, Reich O. Complications and early postoperative outcome after open prostatectomy in patients with benign prostatic enlargement: Results of a prospective multicenter study. The Journal of Urology. 2007;**177**(4):1419-1422

[12] Suer E, Gokce I, Yaman O, Anafarta K, Göğüş O. Open prostatectomy is still a valid option for large prostates: A high-volume, single-center experience. Urology. 2008;**72**(1):90-94

[13] Zargooshi J. Open prostatectomy for benign prostate hyperplasia: Short-term outcome in 3000 consecutive patients. Prostate Cancer and Prostatic Diseases. 2007;**10**:374-377

[14] Tugcu V, Tasci AI, Sahin S, Ordekci Y, Karakas OF, Zorluoglu F. Outcomes of 80 W KTP laser vaporization of the large prostate. Urologia Internationalis 2007;79:316-320

[15] Gunsren KO, Kordan Y, Vuruskan H. Laparoscopic simple prostatectomy. Bulletin of Urooncology. 2014;**13**:215-222. DOI: 10.4274/uob.174

[16] Yuh B, Laungani R, Perlmutter A, Eun D, Peabody JO, Mohler JL, Stricker H, Guru KA. Robot-assisted Millin's retropubic prostatectomy: Case series. The Canadian Journal of Urology. 2008;**15**(3):4101-4105

[17] Stolzenburg J, Kallidonis P, Qazi H, Ho Thi P, Dietel A, Liatsikos EN, Do M. Extraperitoneal approach for robotic-assisted simple prostatectomy. Urology. 2014;**84**:1099-1105

[18] Patel M, Hemal A. Robot-assisted laparoscopic simple anatomic prostatectomy. The Urologic Clinics of North America. 2014;**41**:485-492

[19] Rehman J, Khan SA, Sukkarieh T, Chughtai B, Waltzer WC. Extraperitoneal laparoscopic prostatectomy (adenomectomy) for obstructing benign prostatic hyperplasia: Transvesical and transcapsular (Millin) techniques. Journal of Endourology. 2005; **19**:491-496

[20] Mariano MB, Graziottin TM, Tefilli MV. Laparoscopic prostatectomy with vascular control for benign prostatic hyperplasia. The Journal of Urology. 2002;**167**:2528-2529

[21] Sotelo R, Spaliviero M, Garcia-Segui A, Hasan W, Novoa J, Desai MM, Kaouk JH, Gill IS. Laparoscopic retropubic simple prostatectomy. The Journal of Urology. 2005;**173**: 757-760

[22] van Velthoven R, Peltier A, Laguna MP, Piechaud T. Laparoscopic extraperitoneal adenomectomy (Millin): Pilot study on feasibility. European Urology. 2004;**45**:103-109 discussion 109

[23] Porpiglia F, Terrone C, Renard J, Grande S, Musso F, Cossu M, Vacca F, Scarpa RM. Transcapsular adenomectomy (Millin): A comparative study, extraperitoneal laparoscopy versus open surgery. European Urology. 2006;**49**:120-126

[24] Ellis WJ, Wright JL. Complications of simple prostatectomy. In: Taneja SS, editor. Complications of Urologic Surgery: Prevention and Management. 4th ed. Elsevier; 2010. p. 497-501. https://doi.org/10.1016/B978-1-4160-4572-4.X0001-5

[25] Lucca I, Shariat SF, Hofbauer SL, Klatte T. Outcomes of minimally invasive simple prostatectomy for benign prostatic hyperplasia: A systematic review and meta-analysis. World Journal of Urology. 2015;**33**(4):563-570

[26] Matei DV, Brescia A, Mazzoleni F, Spinelli M, Musi G, Melegari S, Galasso G, Detti S, de Cobelli O. Robot-assisted simple prostatectomy (RASP): Does it make sense? BJU International. 2012;**110**(11 Pt C):E972-E979

[27] Ou R, You M, Tang P, Chen H, Deng X, Xie K. A randomized trial of transvesical prostatectomy versus transurethral resection of the prostate for prostate greater than 80 mL. Urology. 2010;**76**(4):958-961

[28] Parsons JK, Rangarajan SS, Palazzi K, Chang D. A national, comparative analysis of perioperative outcomes of open and minimally invasive simple prostatectomy. Journal of Endourology. 2015;**29**(8):919-924

[29] Tubaro A, Carter S, Hind A, Vicentini C, Miano L. A prospective study of the safety and efficacy of suprapubic transvesical prostatectomy in patients with benign prostatic hyperplasia. The Journal of Urology. 2001;**166**(1):172-176

[30] Varkarakis I, Kyriakakis Z, Delis A, Protogerou V, Deliveliotis C. Long-term results of open transvesical prostatectomy from a contemporary series of patients. Urology. 2004;**64**(2):306-310

[31] Schuessler WW, Schulam PG, Clayman RV, Kavoussi LR. Laparoscopic radical prostatectomy: Initial short-term experience. Urology. 1997;**50**(6):854-857

[32] Baumert H, Ballaro A, Dugardin F, Kaisary AV. Laparoscopic versus open simple prostatectomy: A comparative study. The Journal of Urology. 2006;**175**:1691-1694.24

[33] García-Segui A, Gascón-Mir M. Comparative study between laparoscopic extraperitoneal and open adenomectomy. Actas Urologicas Españolas. 2012;**36**:110-116, 25

[34] McCullough TC, Heldwein FL, Soon SJ, Galiano M, Barret E, Cathelineau X, Prapotnich D, Vallancien G, Rozet F. Laparoscopic versus open simple prostatectomy: An evaluation of morbidity. Journal of Endourology. 2009;**23**:129-133

[35] Nadler RB, Blunt LW Jr, User HM, Vallancien G. Preperitoneal laparoscopic simple prostatectomy. Urology. 2004;**63**:778-779

[36] Rey D, Ducarme G, Hoepffner JL, Staerman F. Laparoscopic adenectomy: A novel technique for managing benign prostatic hyperplasia. BJU International. 2005;**95**:676-678

[37] Mariano MB, Tefilli MV, Graziottin TM, Morales CM, Goldraich IH. Laparoscopic prostatectomy for benign prostatic hyperplasia—A six-year experience. European Urology. 2006;**49**:127-131. discussion 131-2

[38] Hoepffner JL, Gaston R, Piechaud T, Rey D. Finger assisted laparoscopic retropubic prostatectomy (Millin). European Urology Supplements. 2006;**5**:962-967

[39] Oktay B, Vuruskan H, Koc G, Danisoglu ME, Kordan Y. Single-port extraperitoneal transvesical adenomectomy: Initial operative experience. Urologia Internationalis. 2010; **85**:131-134

[40] Chlosta PL, Varkarakis IM, Drewa T, Dobruch J, Jaskulski J, Antoniewicz AA, Borówka A. Extraperitoneal laparoscopic Millin prostatectomy using finger enucleation. The Journal of Urology. 2011;**186**:873-876

Section 6

Simple Prostatectomy Technique - Endoscopic Extraperitoneal Transvesicocapsular Adenomectomy of Prostate

Chapter 6

Endoscopic Extraperitoneal Transvesicocapsular Adenomectomy of Prostate (EETAP): A New Operative Method with an Innovative Learning Protocol for Its Performance

Genadiev Tsvetin Trifonov

Additional information is available at the end of the chapter

http://dx.doi.org/10.5772/intechopen.82225

Abstract

The standard surgical treatment of obstructive symptoms of the lower urinary tract by benign prostatic hyperplasia is transurethral resection or classical simple prostatectomy. Inspired by our experience with laparoscopic radical prostatectomy and for the protection of urethra from stricture during prolonged transurethral resection, we studied the literature and started a prospective study for performing a laparoscopic simple prostatectomy. Following informed patient consent, we performed laparoscopic extraperitoneal simple prostatectomy in 17 patients with moderate to severe obstructive symptoms of benign prostatic hyperplasia with a prostate volume of over 80 ml. We did not find a laparoscopic technique for a simple prostatectomy which is the same as our method that we describe and publish. We called our method endoscopic extraperitoneal transvesicocapsular adenomectomy of prostate. We identified an abbreviation for the method of its popularization and systematic presentation, EETAP. In this chapter, we publish for the first time in the literature a minimally invasive surgical method for endoscopic extraperitoneal transvesicocapsular prostate adenomectomy. We describe and publish the details of the method, the abbreviation of the method, an innovative learning protocol for its performance, as well as hypotheses for preoperative and intraoperative differential diagnosis. In our opinion, a multicenter study of this method could lead to its standardization in the broad urological practice.

Keywords: new minimal invasive operative method, simple prostatectomy, endoscopic extraperitoneal transvesicocapsular adenomectomy, prostate, EETAP, obstructive symptoms of the lower urinary tract, benign prostatic hyperplasia, laparoscopic extraperitoneal simple prostatectomy, innovative learning protocol, preoperative and intraoperative differential diagnosis, urine genetic test, new urine prostate cancer test indications

1. Introduction

For operative treatment of benign prostatic hyperplasia, transurethral resection is used as a standard for prostatic volume up to 75 ml. For larger volumes of the prostate, there is a classic open simple prostatectomy, which we call adenomectomy. The laparoscopic surgical technique was introduced into urology in 1991 with the publication of Schuessler et al. for pelvic lymph node dissection for prostate cancer staging [1]. Shortly thereafter, the first laparoscopic radical prostatectomy published by the same author was performed [2]. The first laparoscopic simple prostatectomy was performed in 1999 by Mariano Mirandolino [3]. In the last 10 years, the laparoscopic surgical technique has been used for the operative treatment of benign prostatic hyperplasia. Various minimally invasive methods for simple prostatectomy performed by laparoscopy are found in the literature. Laparoscopy is performed by transperitoneal access, classical laparoscopy, and extraperitoneal access—endoscopic extraperitoneal technique. A greater number of methods are not described in detail and consistently. Encouraged by our experience with laparoscopic radical prostatectomy and for the protection of the urethra from stricture during prolonged transurethral resection, we started a prospective study to perform and validate endoscopic extraperitoneal surgery for simple prostatectomy in benign prostatic hyperplasia, BPH. We have defined and described the main points of the surgical technique of simple prostatectomy. We present a detailed step-by-step approach to our method. In order to use the experience of a similar laparoscopic method, we compared all the steps of the new method with the previously described surgical technique for endoscopic extraperitoneal radical prostatectomy. We created an innovative protocol for learning and performing the new method based on a comparison of the two surgical methods performed in prostate cancer and prostate adenoma. From this protocol, we built a hypothesis for a new intraoperative approach to suspected carcinoma by express histological examination of the enucleated adenomatous tissue and an assessment of the volume of surgery—radical prostatectomy or adenomectomy. This hypothesis is to be explored. We have also developed a second hypothesis for preoperative differential diagnosis of aggressive prostate cancer by a noninvasive urine test SelectMDx/MDxHealth, Irvine, CA, USA, and Europe, to avoid classical biopsy in selected patients. The role of this hypothesis is related to the presence of 10% incidental cancer in patients after simple prostatectomy, and some authors perform a preoperative classical prostate biopsy on all patients. The indications for urine test performance are limited by the use of 5-alpha-reductase inhibitors as well as in patients with permanent urethral catheter due to inability to spontaneously urinate. However, the method could be used in patients who are candidates for a simple prostatectomy in order to prevent a second operation for incidental prostate cancer. Until now, such indications have not been determined for this urine test.

2. Materials and methods

2.1. Patients

For the period 2014–2017, 17 men, n = 17, of average age 64 years, from 48 to 76, were operated in the Urology Department of Vita Hospital, Sofia, and in the Urology Clinic of Uni

Hospital, City of Panagiurishte. In all, endoscopic extraperitoneal transvesicocapsular adenomectomy of the prostate (EETAP) was done. Preoperative prostate diagnosis was made by PSA total and free, rectal digital prostate examination, transrectal ultrasound, abdominal ultrasound, and flexible urethrocystoscopy. The mean volume of prostate adenoma measured by transrectal ultrasound was 95 ml, 75–140. We performed an evaluation of the international prostate symptom score preoperatively only in patients without residual urine. We have used uroflowmetry in patients with early symptoms of prostate obstruction. Four patients underwent transrectal tru-cut ultrasound prostate biopsy before adenomectomy. We did not have a patient with transurethral resection of the prostate before surgery. All patients signed informed consent for the proposed operation and probability of occlusive prostate cancer despite negative preoperative diagnosis and biopsy. The surgical team has experience in prostate cancer diagnosis and laparoscopic radical prostatectomy. All operations were performed by a single major operator, TTG. This operator is a laparoscopic urologist with experience in endoscopic extraperitoneal radical prostatectomy, experienced in transvesical open simple prostatectomy, but not experienced in open transcapsular Millin adenomectomy.

2.2. Indications

Patients with benign prostatic hyperplasia (BPH), prostate adenoma, and symptoms of obstruction of the lower urinary tract. Prostate volume over 75 ml measured by transrectal ultrasound.

2.3. Contraindications

General contraindications for laparoscopic method—impaired pulmonary and cardiovascular status—as well as those with impaired blood clotting. Patients with a history of a brain accident in the past have been consulting a neurologist to determine the risk of surgery related to Trendelenburg position. Patients with prior inguinal hernioplasty, with or without mesh plastic, have not been contraindicated. Patients with bladder stones or a large prostatic middle lobe are not contraindicated for our method. Asymptomatic uroinfection is not a contraindication to surgery. We do not have pre-treatment and apply a triple antibiotic combination at the beginning of the operation.

3. Operative technique EETAP

In EETAP, preoperative patient preparation, anesthesia, patient's operating table position, operating team position, equipment location in the operating room, type of apparatus and instruments, and position and type of trocars completely coincide with those of endoscopic extraperitoneal radical prostatectomy, EERPE [**Table 1**]. An additional tool is the laparoscopic morcellation device with its own trocar 10 or 12 mm.

3.1. Preoperative patient preparation

Diet regimen, the day before the operation, is as follows: normal daily meals and liquid supper at 18o'clock. Preoperative laxative preparation with suppositories for rectal administration.

	Author/year of publication	Patients, n =	Title name of the method and his abbreviation, if there is, according to the author's publication	Pelvic operative access—trans- or extraperitoneal	Access to adenoma via bladder wall incision, prostatic capsule incision, or vesicocapsular incision	Method of extraction the adenoma from the patient endobag or morcellation
1	Mariano et al., 2002 [3]	1	Laparoscopic prostatectomy with vascular control for benign prostatic hyperplasia	Trans	Midline bladder and capsular incision	Morcellation
2	Nadler et al., 2004 [19]	1	Preperitoneal laparoscopic simple prostatectomy	Extra	Transversal capsular incision	Endobag umbilical extraction
3	van Velthoven et al., 2004 [20]	18	Laparoscopic extraperitoneal adenomectomy (Millin)	Extra	Transversal anterior incision of the prostate capsule	Is not explained
4	Rey et al., 2005 [21]	5	Laparoscopic adenectomy: a novel technique for managing benign prostatic hyperplasia	Extra pre-peritoneal space by a Veress needle	Prostatic capsule is opened 3–4 cm transversally	Laparoscopic bag extracted through the enlarged umbilical incision
5	Sotelo et al., 2005 [22]	17	Laparoscopic simple retropubic prostatectomy	Extra	Transverse cystotomy	Endobag
6	Rehman et al., 2005 [23]	20	Laparoscopic extraperitoneal adenomectomy (LEA)	More than 20	Transversal capsulotomy	Endobag morcellated removed through the subumbilical incision
7	Mariano et al., 2006 [24]	60	Laparoscopic prostatectomy for benign prostatic hyperplasia, a 6-year experience	Extra	Midline incision anterior aspect of the prostatic capsule and bladder neck	Morcellation
8	Porpiglia et al., 2006 [25]	20	Transcapsular adenomectomy (Millin): a comparative study, extraperitoneal laparoscopy versus open surgery	Extra	Transversal capsular incision	Endobag through umbilical port
9	Oktay et al., 2011 [26]	16	Laparoscopic extraperitoneal simple prostatectomy for benign prostate hyperplasia	Extra	Transverse incision at the vesicoprostatic junction of the bladder	Is not explained

	Author/year of publication	Patients, n =	Title name of the method and his abbreviation, if there is, according to the author's publication	Pelvic operative access—trans- or extraperitoneal	Access to adenoma via bladder wall incision, prostatic capsule incision, or vesicocapsular incision	Method of extraction the adenoma from the patient endobag or morcellation
10	Ramón de Fata Chillón et al., 2010 [27]	10	Laparoscopic extraperitoneal adenomectomy	Extra	Vertical capsulotomy from the prostatic apex up to 1 cm above the bladder neck	Laparoscopic bag through the enlarged umbilical incision
11	Yun et al., 2010 [28]	11	Laparoscopic retropubic simple prostatectomy	Extra	Transverse incision of the anterior prostatic capsule	Endobag sac
12	García-Segui and Gascón-Mir, 2012 [29]	28	Laparoscopic extraperitoneal adenomectomy (LEA)	Extra	Transverse incision is made at the vesicoprostatic junction	Endobag sac
13	Xing et al., 2010 [30]	51	Laparoscopic simple prostatectomy with prostatic urethra preservation	Extra	Transverse prostatic capsular incision	Endobag
14	Pedro Romanelli de Castro et al., 2013 [31]	15	Laparoscopic retropubic prostatectomy: initial experience	Ten trans Five extra peritoneal	Opening of the prostate capsule and the bladder neck was made by longitudinal incision	Bagged and removed after morcellation through the umbilical incision
15	Al-Aown, 2015 [32]	11	Laparoscopic simple rostatectomy (LSP)	Extra	3–4 cm vertical cystotomy incision	Endobag
16	Autorino et al., 2015 [18]	843	Minimal invasive simple prostatectomy (MISP)	Extra	Is not explained	Is not explained
17	Garcia-Segu et al., 2015 [33]	26	"Knotless" laparoscopic adenomectomy	Extra	Is not explained	Morcellated adenoma extracted through the umbilical incision
18	Nicoline et al. 2016 [34]	17	Endoscopic transvesical adenomectomy of the prostate (ETAP)	Extraperitoneal but trans vesical percutaneous access	Intravesical bladder incision	Endobag/extraction bag/no data on how exactly to do this

	Author/year of publication	Patients, n =	Title name of the method and his abbreviation, if there is, according to the author's publication	Pelvic operative access—trans- or extraperitoneal	Access to adenoma via bladder wall incision, prostatic capsule incision, or vesicocapsular incision	Method of extraction the adenoma from the patient endobag or morcellation
19	Biktimirov et al., 2017 [35]	79	Minimal invasive simple prostatectomy MISP	Extra	Transverse incision of the anterior prostatic capsule	Removed through the 10 mm port site beneath the umbilicus
20	Baldini et al., 2017 [36]	28	Laparoscopic transcapsular prostatectomy (LTP)	Transperitoneal	Transverse prostatic capsular incision	Is not explained
21	Genadiev TS, 2018 [12]	17	Endoscopic extraperitoneal transvesicocapsular adenomectomy of the prostate (EETAP)	Extra	Transvesicocapsular incision	Morcelation and fragment extraction through the trocar or not morcelated in bag extraction through the left lateral trocar

Extra = extraperitoneal access. Trans = transperitoneal access. Is not explained = there is no explanation of the method in the text.

Table 1. The cited authors on the topic with their main points of the surgical method.

Scheme of administration is as follows: the evening before the surgery at 8 o'clock a suppository and in the morning at 6o'clock before surgery the second suppository. In patients with delayed intestinal passage, we prescribe the oral laxative tablets the day before the operation. Exceptionally, with an unsatisfactory laxative effect, we perform rectal cleansing enema in the morning before the operation. The field of operation is hairless in the evening before the day of surgery. All patients enter the operating room with elastic socks on the legs up to the middle of the thigh. Patients with permanent urethral catheter and urinary tract infections enter the operating room without a catheter. At the beginning of the operation, a combination of antibiotics—cephalosporin, aminoglycoside, and metronidazole—is administered intravenously. In the postoperative period, cephalosporin continues until the patient's discharge, usually 3 days. According to our protocol, prophylaxis with low molecular heparin begins at the sixth hour after the end of the operation. In patients with cardiovascular risk or postoperative bleeding, prophylaxis occurs outside of this protocol.

3.2. Anesthesia

All patients were operated under intubation endotracheal anesthesia with a peripheral venous pathway. Nasogastric tube is not required due to low pressure in the peritoneal cavity in extraperitoneal access. In order to provide free space for the cameramen behind the patient's head, it is necessary to use extended infusion and inhalation systems that distance the anesthesia team and the inhalation device from the patient. A preoperative discussion of the operating time is performed due to the faster onset of hypercapnia in the patient, which is typical for extraperitoneal laparoscopic access. This can be offset by the use of an insufflator with controlled maintenance of the working pressure and dosing of the carbon dioxide flow.

3.3. Position of the patient and operating team

The operating table should have a height of less than 60 cm from the floor level to achieve a good patient operating position and team ergonomics. The patient on the operating table is in the supine position. The hands are fixed to the body. To prevent compartment syndrome and for good blood circulation, the patient's legs remain on the horizontal pads of the operating table without the use of footwell attachments. Also the patient's legs are at the chest level during the Trendelenburg position. The legs remain dissolved at about 30° for access to the rectum, if necessary. At the patient's chest level, a moderately tight belt, 15 cm wide, with a soft pad, is provided to secure the 15° Trendelenburg position—**Figure 1**. Attention is needed against strong chest tightness and difficulty in breathing, as well as against mammary gland trauma.

Location of the operating team—the operator is to the left of the patient, assistant first to the right of the patient, second assistant, and cameramen, behind the patient's head. Surgical nurse is in front of assistant first, to the right of the patient, **Figure 2**.

3.4. Equipment and instruments

Olympus laparoscopic set with automatic insufflator. High-frequency bipolar current generator and ultrasound—Thunderbeat, manufactured by Olympus, Germany, **Figure 3**. Laparoscopic

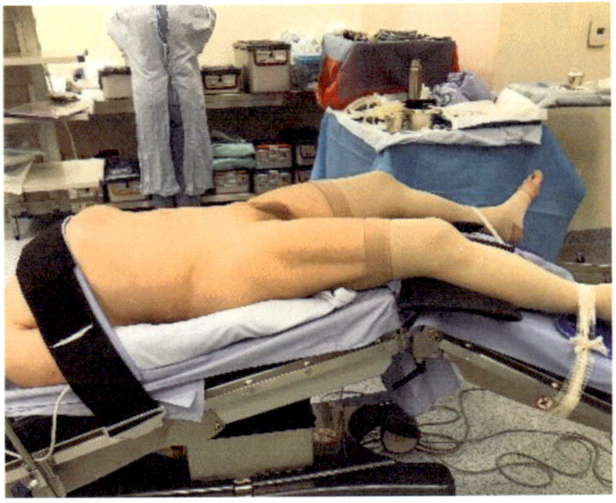

Figure 1. Patient's position on the operative table.

instruments manufactured by Olympus, reusable trocars 5 and 10 mm, Hasson conical trocar 10 mm, and Thunderbeat laparoscopic instrument handle 5 mm, with combined action ultrasonic scissors and bipolar coagulation. Bipolar and traction forceps, needle holders, 5 mm cannula for aspiration, and irrigation with buttons and with piston handle. We do not use any cold scissors during the operation. Stitches are cut with Thunderbeat instrument. The Laparoscope 10 mm with detachable camera head, 0°. Working pressure of carbon dioxide is 12–14 mm mercury. Laparoscopic morcellator devise with 10 mm trocar and grasping forceps 10 mm, manufactured by Richard Wolf, Germany. Morcellation operating speed is 1000 rpm.

The key instruments are Thunderbeat instrument, bipolar forceps, and suction/irrigation 5 mm cannula with pistol handle with two buttons, **Figure 4**.

3.5. Operative access to the pelvis

Operative pelvis access is an endoscopic extraperitoneal balloon dissection of the Retzius space. Performing the pelvic operative field and trocars placement is carried out in a horizontal

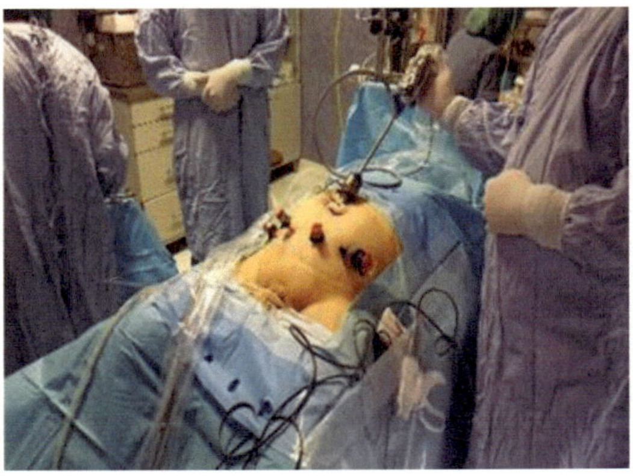

Figure 2. Position of the operating team.

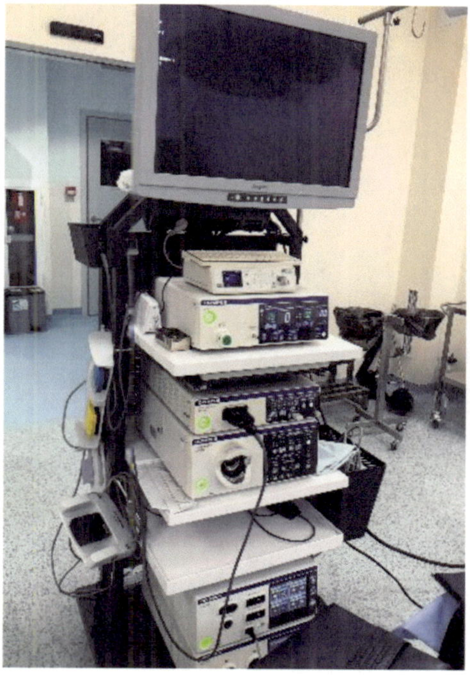

Figure 3. Olympus laparoscopic set with automatic insufflator with high-frequency bipolar current generator with ultrasound source, Thunderbeat, manufactured by Olympus, Germany.

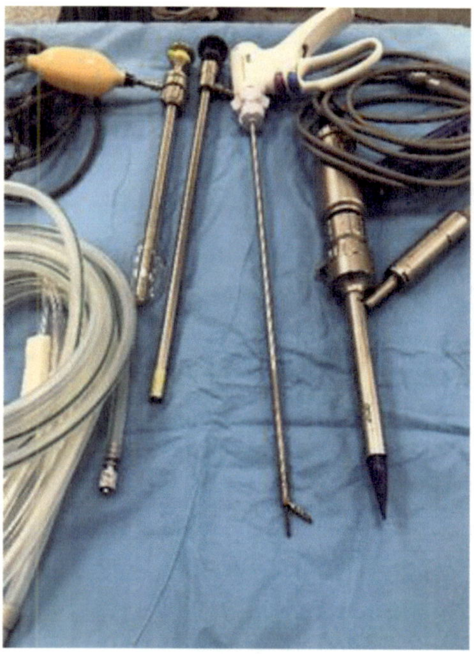

Figure 4. Key instruments: laparoscopic morcellator devise with 10 mm trocar, manufactured by Richard wolf, Germany. Thunderbeat instrument 5 mm, Herloon system for extraperitoneal access.

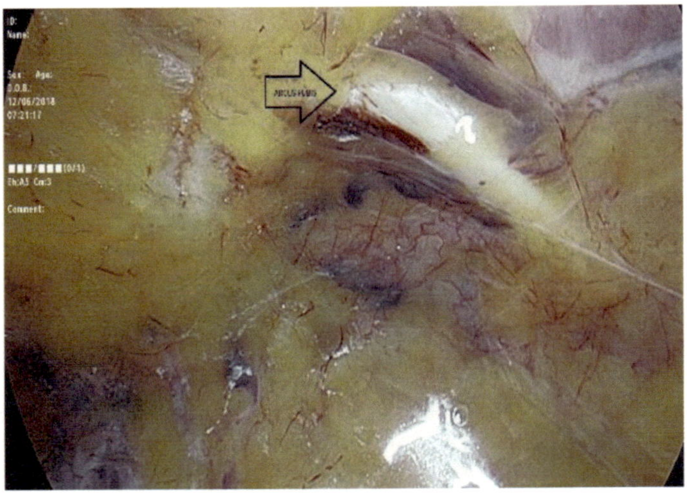

Figure 5. Internal pelvic view through balloon dissector with 10 mm laparoscope shown arcus pubis.

position of the patient to prevent the unnecessary Trendelenburg position. We use balloon dissection device manufactured by Covidien/OMSPDB1000 PDP Round Distension Balloon disposable balloon disposer or by B. Brown or the Herloon System for extraperitoneal access, B. Braun, Aesculap AG, Tuttlingen, Germany. Laparoscopic morcellator devise with 10 mm trocar and grasping forceps 10 mm, manufactured by Richard Wolf, Germany. Approximately 2 cm below the navel is a horizontal 2 cm incision of the skin. The incision site is determined by the depth and width of the pelvis of the patient to ensure good distance of the optic trocar to operative field and against collision with the other trocars. If the patient has a narrow pelvis, then the skin incision can be made slightly to the right of the assistant's side to ensure a good distance between the trocars of the operator. After the skin incision, the fascia of the anterior

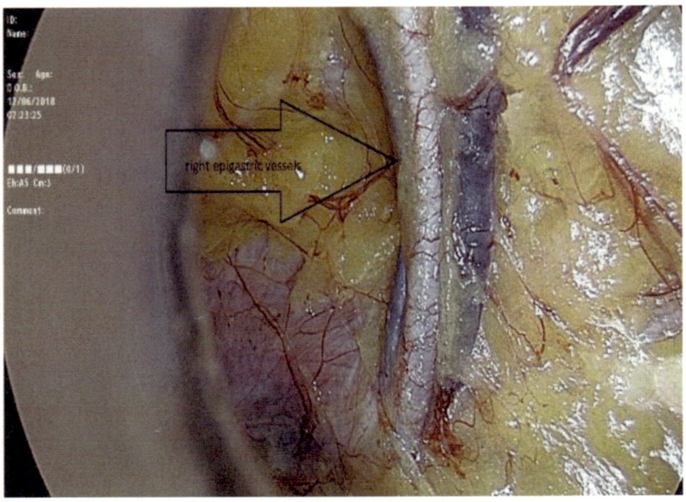

Figure 6. Internal pelvic view through balloon dissector with 10 mm laparoscope shown epigastric vessels.

abdominal wall is reached, which is the anterior fascia of the right abdominal muscles. It is incised transversely about 1–2 cm. Under the fascia, the right abdominal muscles are separated until the peritoneum is detected. Between the peritoneum and the anterior abdominal wall, with the help of the index finger on the right arm, enough space is created for the balloon dissector. The balloon is pumped under visual optical control until the appearance of the pubic arc and the internal epigastric vessels on both sides, **Figures 5** and **6**. After removing the balloon, a Hasson conical trocar is placed and fixed to the abdominal fascia with two slowly absorbable 2/0 Vicryl sutures with "j"-shaped needle, which are finally used to close the fascial insertion. In the case of adhesions of the anterior abdominal wall, which the balloon dissector cannot overcome, the trocars on the opposite side are placed. Adhesion dissection is performed, and access for other trocars is made.

3.6. Trocars: number, type, sequence of placement, and position

The trocars are five. Just the Hasson optical trocar has a smooth surface, because the cone allows to adjust the trocar penetration. Other working trocars must have a spiral surface or accessory fixators to adjust their depth due to the small operative field in the pelvis. Order of placement is as follows: 10 mm cone trocar for laparoscope with adjustable and fixed depth, left side lateral trocar 10 mm with 5 mm reducer, followed by left medial 5 mm, right lateral 5 mm, and right medial 5 mm. Trocars' position is as follows: the two lateral trocars are placed about 2 cm medial from the spina iliaca anterior superior, **Figure 7**. The two medial trocars are placed about 4–5 cm from the lateral ones at a position that provides about 45° of angle between the two working instruments, especially important for inner suturing. These trocars should be placed more cranially for easier suturing of the bladder wall.

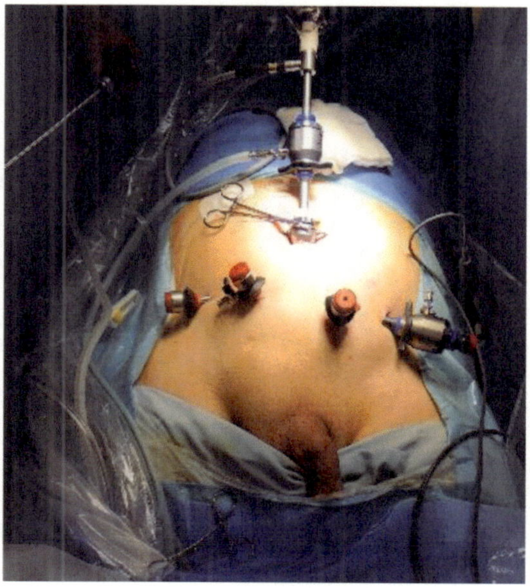

Figure 7. Trocar's position.

4. Operative technique of the inner part of the EETAP

4.1. Incision of the prostatic capsule and bladder neck: transvesicocapsular access to prostate adenoma

Fatty tissue and blood vessels of plexus Santorini are dissected to discovery just the middle surface of the prostatic capsule and the anterior surface of the bladder neck. No hemostatic ligatures on the bladder or capsule are required. The endopelvic fascia, the prostatic ligaments, and dorsal vein complex remain intact. The balloon catheter traction can be used to find bladder neck. The ultrasonic instrument Thunderbeat performs an incision of about 2 cm on the front wall of the bladder in the area of the bladder neck. Immediately after opening the bladder and finding the urethral catheter, the incision continues with the opening of the anterior surface of the bladder neck in the direction of the prostate capsule. Longitudinal incision of the prostatic capsule extends beyond the level of the puboprostatic ligaments to allow good apical dissection and urethral cutting. This is a key point in the EETAP operation and is called transvesicapsular incision, **Figures 8** and **9**.

The advantages of this method are as follows: provides bladder access and inner examination, access to prostate adenoma, good plan for enucleation even in large median lobe, accessibility and good visibility for dissection of the apical part of the urethra without extreme traction of adenoma, good possibilities for bladder trigonisation, large postoperative bladder neck and possibility to avoid trigonisation; spares the inner pelvic anatomy such as dorsal vein complex, puboprostatic ligaments, the prostatovesical pedicles, and the endopelvic fascia to allow conversion to radical prostatectomy if necessary; and allows the same trocars position as EERPE in case of conversion. This method allows good large enucleation plan with prostate capsule preservation from rupturing in the lateral direction where the vascular bundles are located, which is important for our hypothesis of switching to radical prostatectomy during surgery. Last but not least, the transvesicocapsular incision is intuitive to perform and recover for a right-handed surgeon without changing the trocars during inner suturing.

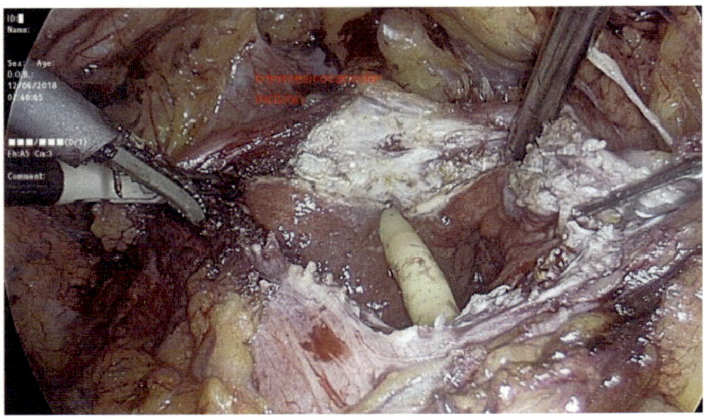

Figure 8. Transvesicocapsular incision—*before* adenoma enucleation. The bladder neck is incised at 12o'clock position longitudinally close to prostatic ligaments. The incision is in deep to the adenoma.

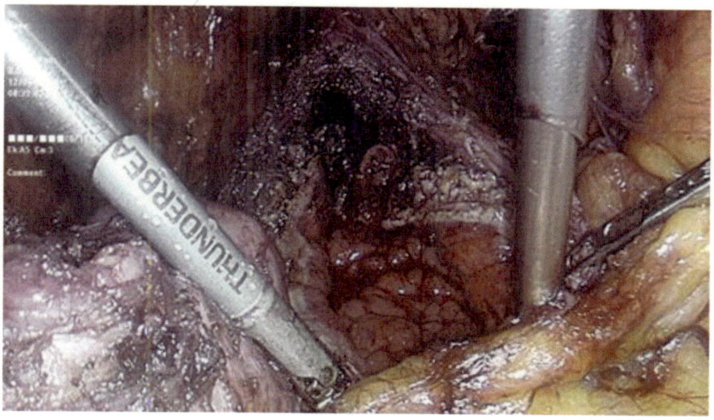

Figure 9. Transvesicocapsular incision—after adenoma enucleation. The prostatic bed is empty. Adenoma is on the left side of the picture.

4.2. Enucleation of adenoma

The enucleation of the adenoma begins with the finding of a plan between the prostate capsule and the adenomatous tissue. This is most often done from the front surface of the bladder neck that is already open to the incision. So if there is a middle prostatic lobe, it does not make it difficult to find a plan. Moreover, if the middle lobe is large, a good plan can be found between its mucosa and the adenoma starting from 6o'clock position of the bladder neck. The enucleation of adenoma is performed by Thunderbeat/Olympus combined with ultrasonic scissors and bipolar coagulation forceps and second bipolar forceps, **Figure 10**. Thus, the bipolar coagulation is possible on the two hands of the operator. With these two instruments, all enucleation is performed without the need for hemostatic ligatures of the internal prostatic pedicles that are coagulated with bipolar forceps. Enucleation is performed under visual control and in a visible manner between the capsule and the adenomatous tissue, following a good and possible plan. If the plan is lost, it goes into another plan. In the case of difficulties in the volume

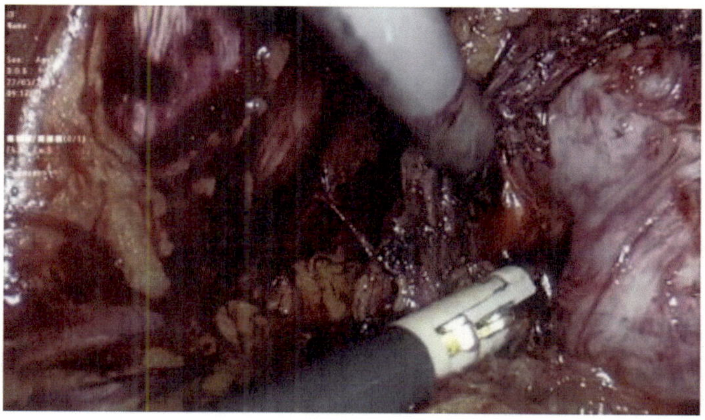

Figure 10. Enucleation plan between capsule and adenoma of the prostate via bipolar forceps and Thunderbeat instrument.

of adenoma, it goes to its division and enucleation of parts. Apical dissection of the urethra requires attention. In this method, this is done with mild or without any traction, and a visible plan to find urethra and colliculus seminalis is to ensure good postoperative urine continence.

4.3. Removing adenoma out of the patient

In our method, removal of the adenoma from the patient is done in two ways. The first method is as follows: a left lateral trocar is extracted and replaced with the laparoscopic morcellator with his own trocar without expanding the trocar hole. The adenoma is morcellating over the prostatic capsule with extraction of the each fragment via grasper immediately after his own morcellation. Beware of residual fragments in the bladder and on the pelvic wall! At the end of the morcellation, a revision of residual fragments is performed. The morcellator is pulled out under optics control, and the working trocar is reinserted, **Figure 11**.

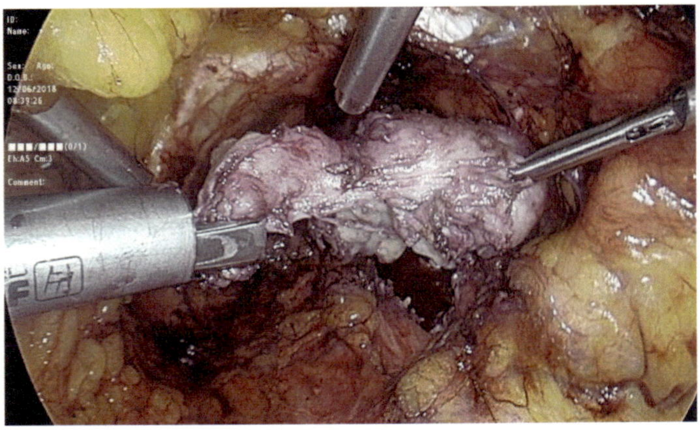

Figure 11. Morcellation of the adenoma. The morsellator is placed through the left lateral trocar hole without skin extension.

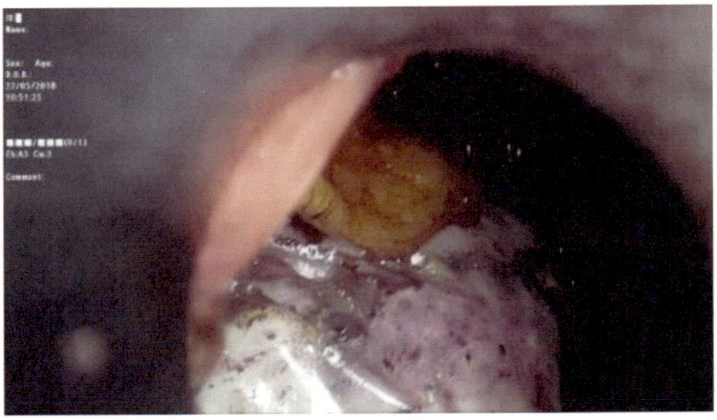

Figure 12. Enucleated adenoma in endobag and fixed through the left lateral trocar hole. The endobag can be extracted for histology examination.

http://dx.doi.org/10.5772/intechopen.82225

The second method is as follows: after complete release of the adenoma, it is placed in an endobag/sterile laparoscopic plastic bag that is fixed around the left lateral trocar and remains thus until the end of the inner part of the operation, **Figure 12**. This method is the same as in EERPE technique and allows extracting adenoma for an express histology test for cancer during the operation. If not necessary, then at the end of the operation, the left lateral trocar is removed, and his opening widens, and the endobag is removed through it. In order not to extend the trocar hole too far, the adenoma is subdivided by ultrasonic scissors into smaller fragments within the endobag. The removed material is fixed in formalin for a histological preparation.

4.4. Closure of the transvesicocapsular incision

Prostatic bed hemostasis is performed with bipolar coagulation at reduced working pressure of carbon dioxide up to 8 mm mercury. After hemostasis of the prostatic bed, 3-0/Monocryl™ Plus, MCP 4160, Ethicon®, needle 1/2c, 26 mm, and Johnson and Johnson; hemostatic sutures of the bladder neck on the 5 and 7o'clock position are made, and suturing the trigonum as close as possible to the urethra is performed. This is the so-called trigonisation, **Figure 13**. Following trigonisation, a three-way 22 charier catheter is inserted in the urethra to the bladder. The incision of the prostate and bladder wall is restored with continuous suture 2-0 monocryl/Vicryl™, Ethicon®, Johnson and Johnson, W9121, 26 mm, 1/2c needle, **Figure 14**. The suture starts from the apical part of the prostatic capsule and continues to the bladder wall up to the end of incision. Care should be taken not to suture the catheter. At the end of suturing, the catheter is checked for mobility. Then the balloon is placed sure in the bladder and inflated with 60 ml saline. Verification of the bladder for leakage, and start the irrigation through the catheter. Place a 14–16 charier tube drainage through a right lateral trocar hole. The skin of the trocar holes is closed with tissue glue/Hystoacryl® 0.5 ml, B. Braun Surgical, S.A./except for the hole in the tube drain. In this method the bladder neck inside remains open, with the suture engaging only the front of the bladder wall. Thus, we believe that a broad bladder-to-prostate communication is created to prevent post-operative bladder neck

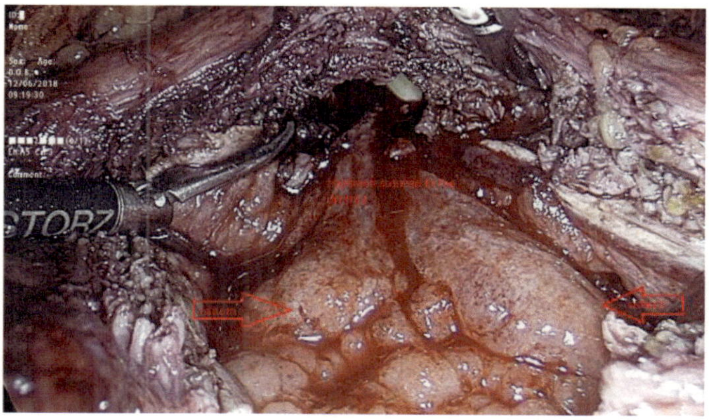

Figure 13. Bladder trigonisation. The wide bladder neck remains open after incision closure.

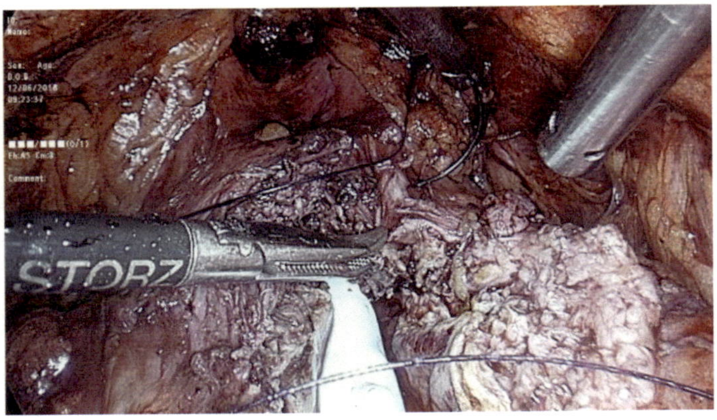

Figure 14. Closure of the transvesicocapsular incision with 2/0 Monocryl continuous suture over the urethral catheter.

sclerosis. Furthermore, this extensive communication does not make trigonisation mandatory if there are technical difficulties to do so.

4.5. Postoperative protocol

Our postoperative recovery protocol for EETAP is the same as our EERPE protocol. The only difference is the catheter irrigation after adenomectomy. This recovery protocol has the following steps: 6 hours after anesthesia, the patient is under monitoring, moves up, and takes fluids at the end of the sixth hour after the end of anesthesia. Thirty minutes before the movement, a subcutaneous application of low molecular heparin was administered. The irrigation of the catheter is stopped the next day, which is the first postoperative day. The balloon of the catheter remains inflated till the cystography. On a second or third postoperative day, the patient leaves the clinic. Ambulatory therapy for a total of 10 days with antibiotic per oral and prophylaxis with low molecular heparin is used. After the sixth postoperative day, cystography is performed in the ambulatory, and the urethral catheter is removed. We monitor and interview the patient monthly for urinary infection and sclerosis of the bladder neck until the third postoperative month.

5. Results

Average operative time skin to skin was 150 minutes (from 90 to 180). Average catheter stay was 7 days/6–9 days. There was no case of blood transfusions. There was no case of operative conversion or postoperative open or laparoscopic revision. There was no case of major complication such as vessel thrombosis or postoperative death. There was one case of early postoperative transurethral revision due to hematuria but without prolonged catheter stay and blood transfusion. The our second patient, who had the 140 ml prostate, mainly with big median lobe, required transurethral resection on the third month after EETAP due to the large prostatic residual tissue on both sides. In fact we had removal just the big middle lobe. One patient reports stress incontinence until 6 postoperative months. Without patients with new catheterization due to urinary retention. None of the patients reported impaired erectile function or full urine incontinence. There are five cases of subdermal hematomas, typical after extraperitoneal access. Preoperative prostate biopsy was performed in four patients. We did not have a case with accidentally exposed prostate cancer. All patients reported satisfaction with the first urination after catheter removal. From our postoperative observation and patient interview to 90 postoperative day, we did not have a patient with bladder neck sclerosis, bladder stones, or other urological postoperative complications.

6. Discussion

Our laparoscopic practice began in 2003 with our first laparoscopic staging lymph node dissection in prostate cancer [4]. In 2005 we introduced in our practice the Montsouris technique of transperitoneal radical prostatectomy [5, 6]. Three years later we start to perform the endoscopic extraperitoneal radical prostatectomy technique described by Stolzenburg et al., [7, 8]. We published a new endoscopic extraperitoneal method for bladder stones in 2011 [9]. In our diagnostic practice, we introduced the transrectal ultrasound tru-cut prostate biopsy in 2004 [10], the ratio of free to total PSA in 2005 [11], and urine test SelectMDx in 2017 [12]. These circumstances and the protection of the urethra from prolonged transurethral resection motivated us to carry out and validate the new EETAP method. For exploring and describing our method, we were guided by the main points of our technique—surgical access, access to the prostate capsule and adenoma, a method of removing adenoma from the patient. We only discuss sources and authors that are closely related to the keywords of our method. Authors describing laparoscopic robot-assisted, single-port, hybrid, and operative techniques other than our method are not discussed here.

According to the Guidelines of European Association of Urology, the term minimal invasive simple prostatectomy (MISP) includes laparoscopic simple prostatectomy (LSP) and robot-assisted simple prostatectomy (RASP) [13]. Both methods are based on the transcapsular (Millin) or transvesical (Freyer) techniques. According to Guidelines of American Urological Association, the methods with minimal invasion are called minimally invasive surgical therapies, MIST. There is no abbreviation for laparoscopic simple prostatectomy [14]. According to Canadian UA Guideline 2010 Update: Guidelines for the Management of Benign Prostatic Hyperplasia, minimally invasive surgical therapies (MIST), and in the open simple prostatectomy section, there is no word laparoscopy or other laparoscopic simple prostatectomies. No current data from the Canadian urologist association are available on this topic [15].

Sequence of stages and their steps	Surgical technique step by step	EERPE Prostate cancer Stages and steps	EETAP Prostate adenoma Stages and steps	Match between EERPE and EETAP
First stage in seven steps: preoperative and operative preparation				
1	Preoperative patient preparation	Yes	Yes	Match
2	Operating team	Yes	Yes	Match
3	Position of team in the operating room	Yes	Yes	Match
4	Patient table position	Yes	Yes	Match
5	Trendelenburg position	Yes	Yes	Match
6	Equipment	Yes	Yes	Match
7	Instrumental equipment	Yes	Yes	Match
Second stage in four steps: operative access				
8	Pelvic endoscopic access via balloon dissection	Yes	Yes	Match
9	Trocars: numbers and kinds	Yes	Yes	Match
10	Trocar position	Yes	Yes	Match
11	Access to the prostatic surface	Yes	Yes	Match
Stage three in seven steps: intracorporal part of both operative techniques				
12	Endopelvic fascia incision	Yes	No	Matchless
13	Ligation of the dorsal vessels of the penis	Yes	No	Matchless
14	Longitudinal transvesicocapsular incision of the prostate capsule and bladder neck	No	Yes	Matchless
15	Interruption of the bladder neck	Yes	No	Matchless
16	Enucleation of prostatic adenoma	No	Yes	Matchless
17	Prostatovesiculectomy	Yes	No	Matchless
18	Urethrovesical anastomosis	Yes	No	Matchless
Stage four in five steps: final steps of the operations				
19	Removal of operative tissue via morcellation	No	Yes	Matchless
20	Lymph node dissection	Yes	No	Matchless

Sequence of stages and their steps	Surgical technique step by step	EERPE Prostate cancer Stages and steps	EETAP Prostate adenoma Stages and steps	Match between EERPE and EETAP
21	Removal tissue via endobag extraction	Yes	Yes	Match
22	Inner suture	Yes	Yes	Match
23	Kind of suture materials	Yes	Yes	Match
24	Trocars hole closure	Yes	Yes	Match
Stage five in three steps: postoperative protocol				
25	Postoperative recovery period/ catheter irrigation mentioned	Yes	Yes	Match
26	Patient discharge on POD 3–4	Yes	Yes	Match
27	Cystography on POD 5–7	Yes	Yes	Match
Steps number, 27		**24/3**	**21/6**	
Steps matching/correlation ratio, yes/no				

Both techniques in this protocol are presented with the same full steps, 27, and the same stages, 5. EERPE and EETAP are comparable and matching them in almost complete. Endobag = laparoscopic plastic bag.

Table 2. This table presents the innovative learning protocol based on matching according to the main stages and the individual steps for each of the both operative techniques—EERPE and EETAP.

According to Tagard, transvesicocapsular adenomectomy was first described in 1948 by Ogier Ward, later from Bourque in 1954 and Watss in 1956 [16]. In this method, the prostatic capsule and bladder neck are open longitudinally. We have appreciated this and have adopted this method as a key and fundamental feature in our new operating technique.

Historically the first laparoscopic radical prostatectomy was performed and published by Schuessler et al. [2]. According to Delgado-Guerrero, 2016, the first case of laparoscopic simple prostatectomy, adenomectomy, was published by Dr. Mariano Mirandolino, who in 1999 performed the first adenomectomy of a 71-year-old man in Brazil through an extraperitoneal longitudinal incision of the prostate capsule [17]. Dr. Mariano Mirandolino is the pioneer of this operation. He published his 60 operated patients, but he did not describe the surgical technique in detail [24]. Autorino et al. published results from multicenter study and summarized that the laparoscopic simple prostatectomy was performed using different personal techniques developed based on the principles of transcapsular (Millin), transvesical (Freyer), or transvesicocapsular (Bourque) techniques, described for open simple prostatectomy. The same author said that each investigator adopted specific operative strategies and technical moments to optimize this procedure [18]. We completely agree with this after our study of the literature on this topic. We find a lot of author's papers who present the simple prostatectomy on the principles of laparoscopy. They mainly describe the indications and results of the method without providing a detailed description of the surgical technique and the significance of each stage of it. We have not found another description of a laparoscopic method for simple prostatectomy that coincides with ours.

Obviously the laparoscopic simple prostatectomy is not difficult for an experienced laparoscopic urologist. More of cited authors mentioned their laparoscopic radical prostatectomy experience. From a review of literature, it can be seen that laparoscopic radical prostatectomy and laparoscopic simple prostatectomy began their development together [2, 3]. Probably due to standardized transurethral monopolar resection and classical open simple prostatectomy, laparoscopic simple prostatectomy develops more slowly. However, the lack of a consistent description of the details of the method does not allow it to be used for comparative training. The study of many different methods does not allow to create a true value and to standardize one of them. We classified the publications closest to our method according to the benchmarks of the operating technique, as it is shown in **Table 1**.

Therefore, we accept that operative methods published by other authors cannot serve for training. That is why we have decided to describe our new method in detail by comparing it to a similar one in prostate cancer, which is widely used, endoscopic extraperitoneal radical prostatectomy (EERPE) [8]. We have not found another description of a laparoscopic method for simple prostatectomy that coincides with ours. There is one method with abbreviation similar to ours but in fact is completely different [34]. So we did an innovative learning protocol. This protocol compares the EERPE surgical procedure to our adenomectomy surgical technique, EETAP. Moreover, training protocols for endoscopic extraperitoneal radical prostatectomy are found in the literature that can serve to build operator skills as a basis for our method [37–39]. According to the learning protocol of Stolzenburg JU, even residents without open surgery skills can perform EERPE after learning this protocol [40]. Thus, the operator's skills for one method can be applied to the other method, as shown in **Table 2**. Through it we believe that it is possible to introduce and standardize our method in practice.

The correlation ratio in **Table 2** between the two techniques shows that the skills for EREPE can be the basis for implementing EETAP. Moreover, this confirms our hypothesis for intraoperative conversion of adenomectomy into radical prostatectomy, if necessary. Mariano et al., 2006, reported a prostate biopsy in all 60 patients before being operated by laparoscopic simple prostatectomy [24]. Van Velthoven et al. [20], published in 11% of the operated patient's prostate cancer and three high-grade pin [26]. We have done prostate biopsy to four of our patients. Fortunately, we do not have a postoperative prostate cancer patient. None of the authors described behavior in patients with postoperative prostate cancer. Are they performing a second operation or applying another method? We assume that our hypothesis for an intraoperative solution based on express histological examination in selected cases can solve this problem. The disadvantage of this hypothesis is the absence of a pathological preoperative stage, as is achieved in the puncture prostate biopsy. We also offer a second hypothesis for preoperative differential diagnosis of prostate cancer suspected patients by performing a noninvasive urine test SelectMDx [41, 42]. This test is popular as a liquid biopsy because of its high negative predictive value for aggressive prostate cancer with Gleason score of 7 to 10. The test is recommended of prostate cancer diagnosis in the European Urological Guidelines for 2018 [43]. We introduced this test in our daily practice since November 2017 [12]. The negative predictive value of the test is 98% for prostate cancer Gleason score 7, 99% for Gleason scores 8–10. Thus, this test can be the modern solution for preoperative diagnosis. Via SelectMDx test, patients who are candidates for BPH surgery can minimize incidental cancer to 8% or less and could replace the preoperative classical prostate biopsy. We cannot prove this hypothesis at this new indication due to lack of enough cases from our practice. However, this new hypothesis may be the basis for a prospective study to determine a new indication for this urine test. Patients receiving 5-alpha reductase inhibitors as well as those with a permanent urethral catheter are contraindicated or not be able to this method.

7. Conclusion

The operative treatment of urinary symptoms of benign enlarged prostate is performed with the main purpose of achieving satisfactory spontaneous urination for the patient. Our main motive is to find and describe a surgical method that protects the urethra from damage and brings to the patient the benefits of the open simple prostatectomy without its complications. Various surgical techniques for laparoscopic simple prostatectomy are found in the literature. Published cases are a bit about world practice. The world's largest urological recommendations do not define a proven method for laparoscopic simple prostatectomy. There is no detailed description of a method to be adopted and standardized. For the first time in the literature, a surgical method of endoscopic extraperitoneal transvesicocapsular adenomectomy of the prostate (EETAP) is discussed and published. This method may be performed by an operator with experience in endoscopic extraperitoneal radical prostatectomy according to our innovative learning protocol in this respect. In our opinion, this new method, its detailed description, its abbreviation, the innovative protocol for its application, and the new diagnostic hypotheses can serve as a basis for multicenter studies and conclusions for its standardization in the broad urological practice.

Conflict of interest

The author declares no conflict of interest.

Author details

Genadiev Tsvetin Trifonov

Address all correspondence to: genadievi@abv.bg

Department of Urology, Vita Hospital, Sofia, Bulgaria

References

[1] Schuessler WW, Vancaillie TG, Reich H, Griffith DP. Transperitoneal endosurgical lymphadenectomy in patients with localized prostate cancer. The Journal of Urology. 1991;**145**(5):988-991

[2] Schuessler WW, Kavoussi LR, Clayman RV, Vancaille TH. Laparoscopic radical prostatectomy: Initial case report. The Journal of Urology. 1992;**147**:246A

[3] Mariano MB, Graziottin TM, Tefilli MV. Laparoscopic prostatectomy with vascular control for benign prostatic hyperplasia. The Journal of Urology. 2002;**167**(6):2528-2529

[4] Tsvetin G. Laparoscopic pelvic lymph dissection—First results. Oncologos. 2003;**4**:42-47. In Bulgarian

[5] Guillonneau B, Vallancien G. Laparoscopic radical prostatectomy: The Montsouris experience. The Journal of Urology. 2000;**163**:418-422

[6] Genadiev Tsvetin TR. Laparoscopic radical prostatectomy: Initial 22 cases in Bulgarian urological practice. Acta Medica Bulgarica. 2008;**1**:43-46

[7] Genadiev Tsvetin TR, Gaidarov D, Veleva V. Endoscopic extraperitoneal radical prostatectomy—First results. Uronet. 2009;**1**:5-7. In Bulgarian

[8] Stolzenburg JU, Do M, Pfeiffer H, König F, Aedtner B, Dorschner W. The endoscopic extraperitoneal radical prostatectomy (EERPE): Technique and initial experience. World Journal of Urology. 2002;**20**(1):48-55

[9] Genadiev Tsvetin TR. In: Meinhold-Heerlein I, editor. Laparoscopic Extraperitoneal Approach for Urinary Bladder Stones Removal—A New Operative Technique, Laparoscopy—An Interdisciplinary Approach. Rijeka, Croatia: InTech; 2011

[10] Genadiev Tsvetin TR. Transrectal puncture biopsy of the prostate. Urology. 2004;**10**:3, 71-74. In Bulgarian

[11] Boncheva M, Genadiev Tsvetin TR, Petrov P, Halachev N, Gaidarov D, Nakov E. Diagnostic sensitivity and diagnostic specificity of the PSA ratio. Medinfo. 2005;**7**:9-10. In Bulgarian

[12] Genadiev Tsvetin TR, Hristov C, Gaidarov D. Urine genetic test SelectMDx for prostate cancer diagnosis—Initial clinical experience. GP News. 2018;**6**(216):24-26. In Bulgarian

[13] http://uroweb.org/guideline/treatment-of-non-neurogenic-male-luts/#5

[14] http://auanet.org/guidelines/benign-prostatic-hyperplasia/lower-urinary-tract-symptoms-(2018)#x8196

[15] https://www.cua.org/en/guidelines

[16] Tagart REB. Prostatectomy by the vesico-capsular method. British Medical Journal. 1961;**4**:621-626

[17] Delgado-Guerreroa F, Covarrubias-Méndeza LM, González-Gómezb A, Bernal Hernándezb J, Torres-Aguilara J, Arellano-Cuadrosa R. Experience with laparoscopic prostatic adenomectomy. Revista Mexicana de Urología. 2016;**76**(1):17-22

[18] Autorino R, Zargar H, Mariano MB, Sanchez-Salas R, et al. Perioperative outcomes of robotic and laparoscopic simple prostatectomy: A European-American multi-institutional analysis. European Urology. 2015;**68**(1):86-94

[19] Nadler RB, Blunt LW Jr, User HM, Vallancien G. Preperitoneal laparoscopic simple prostatectomy. Urology. 2004;**63**(4):778-779

[20] Van Velthoven R, Peltier A, Laguna MP, Piechaud T. Laparoscopic extraperitoneal adenomectomy (Millin): Pilot study on feasibility. European Urology. 2004;**45**(1):103-109

[21] Rey D, Ducarme G, Hoepffner JL, Staerman F. Laparoscopic adenectomy: A novel technique for managing benign prostatic hyperplasia. BJU International. 2005;**95**(4):676-678

[22] Sotelo R, Spaliviero M, Garcia-Segui A, Hasan W, Novoa J, Desai MM, et al. Laparoscopic retropubic simple prostatectomy. The Journal of Urology. 2005;**173**(3):757-760

[23] Rehman J, Khan SA, Sukkarieh T, Chughtai B, Waltzer WC. Extraperitoneal laparoscopic prostatectomy (adenomectomy) for obstructing benign prostatic hyperplasia: Transvesical and transcapsular (Millin) techniques. Journal of Endourology. 2005;**19**(4):491-496

[24] Mariano MB, Tefilli MV, Graziottin TM, Morales CM, Goldraich IH. Laparoscopic prostatectomy for benign prostatic hyperplasia—A six-year experience. European Urology. 2006;**49**(1):127-131

[25] Porpiglia F, Terrone C, Renard J, Grande S, Musso F, Cossu M, et al. Transcapsular adenomectomy (Millin): A comparative study, extraperitoneal laparoscopy versus open surgery. European Urology. 2006;**49**(1):120-126

[26] Oktay B, Koc G, Vuruskan H, Danisoglu ME, Kordan Y. Laparoscopic extraperitoneal simple prostatectomy for benign prostate hyperplasia: A two-year experience. Urology Journal. 2011;**8**(2):107-112

[27] Ramón de Fata Chillón F, Nuñez Mora C, García Mediero JM, Cabrera Castillo P, García Tello A, Angulo Cuesta J. Laparoscopic extraperitoneal adenomectomy: Surgical technique and preliminary results. Actas Urologicas Españolas. 2010;**34**(9):806-810

[28] Yun HK, Kwon JB, Cho SR, Kim JS. Early experience with laparoscopic retropubic simple prostatectomy in patients with voluminous benign prostatic hyperplasia (BPH). Korean Journal of Urology. 2010;**51**(5):323-329

[29] García-Segui A, Gascón-Mir M. Comparative study between laparoscopic extraperitoneal and open adenomectomy. Actas Urologicas Españolas. 2012;**36**(2):110-116

[30] Xing N, Guo Y, Yang F, Tian L, Zhang J, Yan Y, et al. Laparoscopic simple prostatectomy with prostatic urethra preservation for benign prostatic hyperplasia. Translational Andrology and Urology. 2012;**1**(1):9-13

[31] de Castro PR, Nishimoto RH, Pinheiro RGÂ, Arantes PB d O, Issa AMN, Issa HMN. Laparoscopic retropubic prostatectomy: Initial experience. Revista Médica de Minas Gerais. 2013;**23**(2):178-181

[32] Al-Aown A, Liatsikos E, Panagopoulos V, Kyriazis I, Kallidonis P, Georgiopoulos I, et al. Laparoscopic simple prostatectomy: A reasonable option for large prostatic adenomas. Urology Annals. 2015;**7**(3):297-302

[33] Garcia-Segui A, Verges A, Galán-Llopis JA, Garcia-Tello A, Ramón de Fata F, Angulo JC. "Knotless" laparoscopic extraperitoneal adenomectomy. Actas Urologicas Españolas. 2015;**39**(2):128-136

[34] Kil NMP, Fossion LMCL. Endoscopische transvesicale adenomectomie van de prostaat (ETAP). Resultaten van de eerste 17 patiënten in een perifeerziekenhuis. Tijdschrift voor Urologie. 2016;**6**:104-112

[35] Biktimirov RG, Martov AG, Biktimirov TR, Kaputovskii AA. The role of extraperitoneoscopic adenomectomy in the management of benign prostatic hyperplasia greater than 80 cm^3. Urologiia. 2017;(6):76-81

[36] Baldini A, Fassi-Fehri H, Duarte RC, Crouzet S, Ecochard R, Abid N, et al. Holmium laser enucleation of the prostate versus laparoscopic transcapsular prostatectomy: Perioperative results and three-month follow-up. Current Urology. 2017;**10**(2):81-86. DOI: 10.1159/000447156

[37] Tobias-Machado M, Pazeto CL, Neves-Neto OC, Nunes-Silva I, Zampolli HC. A safe teaching protocol of LRP (laparoscopic radical prostatectomy). International Brazilian Journal of Urology. 2018;**44**(2):273-279

[38] Klein J, Teber D, Frede T, Stock C, Hruza M, Gözen A, et al. Development, validation and operating room-transfer of a six-step laparoscopic training program for the vesicourethral anastomosis. Journal of Endourology. 2013;**27**(3):349-354

[39] Stolzenburg JU, Schwaibold H, Bhanot SM, Rabenalt R, Do M, Truss M, et al. Modular surgical training for endoscopic extraperitoneal radical prostatectomy. BJU International. 2005;**96**(7):1022-1027

[40] Stolzenburg JU, Rabenalt R, Do M, Horn LC, Liatsikos EN. Modular training for residents with no prior experience with open pelvic surgery in endoscopic extraperitoneal radical prostatectomy. European Urology. 2006;**49**(3):491-498

[41] https://mdxhealth.com/company-overview

[42] Leyten GH et al. Identification of a candidate gene panel for the early diagnosis of prostate cancer. Clinical Cancer Research. 2015;**21**(13):3061-3070

[43] https://uroweb.org/guideline/prostate-cancer/#5

Section 7

Radical Prostatectomy Technique - Reduced Port Laparoscopic Prostatectomy

Chapter 7

Reduced Port Extraperitoneal Laparoscopic Radical Prostatectomy

Kazuhiro Araki and Yukio Naya

Additional information is available at the end of the chapter

http://dx.doi.org/10.5772/intechopen.79364

Abstract

Robot-assisted laparoscopic prostatectomy (RALP) is more popular than laparoscopic radical prostatectomy (LRP) in twenty-first century. However, RALP is still an expensive surgery. Open radical prostatectomy (ORP) was a gold standard and not an expensive surgery. However, ORP is not minimum invasive. LRP is relative expensive and minimum invasive. The problem of RALP or LRP is necessary to spread the wound for removing prostate and the pain of wound is often a problem. Using U-shaped incision at umbilicus, spreading the wound is not necessary to remove prostate. Single-port surgery is a challenging procedure for surgeons in spite of faster recovery and higher patient satisfaction than conventional laparoscopy. Adding one or two port, reduced port surgery is easier than single-port surgery. Reduced port LRP is an extension of conventional LRP. The procedure is as same as conventional LRP. Curved or flexible instruments are not always necessary in the reduced port LRP. Reduced port LRP has less pain and better cosmetics than conventional LRP because the prostate is removed from the umbilicus. It is not necessary to spread the wound for removing prostate.

Keywords: reduced port LRP, conventional LRP, umbilicus, EZ access

1. Introduction

Nowadays, robot-assisted laparoscopic prostatectomy (RALP) is more popular than laparoscopic prostatectomy (LRP). However, RALP is a most expensive surgery. The overall cost consequence of RALP was estimated at an additional €2459 (95% CI 1377–3540, p = 0.003) as compared with ORP and an additional €3860 (95% CI 559–7160, p = 0.031) as compared with LRP [1]. Rabenalt et al. reported single-port LRP in 2010 and Amin et al. and Cáceres et al., reported in 2011 and 2012 [2–4]. Single-port surgery leaves little to no scarring and may reduce complications that commonly occur after traditional open and even traditional laparoscopic abdominal surgery. Patients are reporting less discomfort and faster recovery compared with those undergoing traditional laparoscopy. Tugcu et al. reported that single-port pyeloplasty can offer faster recovery and higher patient satisfaction than conventional laparoscopic pyeloplasty [5].

Ca'ceres et al. reported their 31 case of single-port LRP. In their results, mean operative time was 207 min and mean estimated blood loss was 258 ml. The average length of stay was 2.9 days and visual analog pain score (range: 0 [no pain] to 10) at day 2 was 1.2. Five focal positive margins (16.7%) were encountered. Major complications occurred in two patients (6.5%) (hypercapnia with respiratory acidosis and rectourethral fistula) and minor complications in four (12.9%) (atrial fibrillation, orchitis, transfusion, and vomiting). No case required additional analgesia. Thus, single-port LRP might be a safe procedure for skillful surgeon. However, for common surgeons, the single-port approach is more challenging than traditional laparoscopy because the surgeon has less freedom of movement with all instruments using the same entry point. Specially designed flexible instruments help to overcome that limitation. Sato et al. reported that 469 single-site surgeries were carried out between February 2009 and December 2012 at nine academic institutions in Japan. Radical prostatectomy was carried out in only six cases [6].

However, adding one or two port, reduced port surgery is easier than single-port surgery. Reduced port LRP is an extension of conventional LRP. The procedure is as same as conventional LRP. Recently, we perform several reduced port laparoscopic surgery, such as pyeloplasty, partial nephrectomy, excision of urachal remnant, and prostatectomy. We start reduced port LRP from April 2018. In this chapter, we introduce reduced port LRP. Reduced port LRP has less pain and better cosmetics than conventional LRP. It is not necessary to spread the wound for removing prostate.

2. Reduced port LRP

2.1. Indications

Radical prostatectomy (RP) is an appropriate therapy for any patients with clinically localized prostate cancer that can be completely excised surgically, who has a life expectancy of 10 years and more and has no serious conditions that would contraindicate an elective operation.

The indications for laparoscopic RP (LRP) are same as that of open radical prostatectomy.

Absolute contraindications to laparoscopic prostatectomy include the inability to undergo general anesthesia or uncorrectable bleeding diatheses.

Patients who had a history of inguinal mesh herniorrhaphy, or primary transurethral resection of prostate (TURP) 3–4 months before LRP, is not an indication of extraperitoneal LRP. Inguinal hernia repair with the incorporation of prosthetic mesh has been reported to create a dense, fibrotic reaction, complicating future pelvic procedures [7]. There have been several reports of surgeons encountering severe fibrosis and scarring during RRP in patients who have undergone prior mesh hernia repairs, leading to early termination of the procedure [8–10]. Recent several studies have reported that transperitoneal LRP after prior laparoscopic inguinal herniorrhaphy is feasible and does not adversely affect operative and functional results [11–13]. In my experience, adhesions and distortion of normal anatomy is a serious problem of performed extraperitoneal prostatectomy. It is better to consider transperitoneal approach.

Capsular perforation during TURP and extravasation of the irrigation fluid might be periprostatic fibrosis. Fibrosis of the previously resected bladder neck may lead to worse healing at the anastomosis [14, 15]. Menard et al. compare the morbidity and functional results after laparoscopic radical prostatectomy with and without previous TURP [16]. They performed LRP at least 3 months after TURP. They concluded LRP after TURP can be performed without compromising the radical nature of cancer surgery. However, the procedure is associated with worse intraoperative and postoperative outcomes with respect to operative time, length of catheter stay, length of hospital stay, and surgical complication rate. Gellhaus et al. reported the results of RALP after HoLEP. According to their report, the posterior bladder neck and apical dissections were significantly more challenging in the setting of previous HoLEP [17].

2.2. Informed consent

As with open surgery, patients must be counseled on the risk of adjacent organ injury, such as ureter, rectum, bladder, and iliac vessels. Patients undergoing LRP must be aware of the potential for open conversion. The risk of general anesthesia should be presented to the patients.

2.3. Bowel preparation

Considering the risk of rectum injury, a preoperative bowel preparation may be used. The patient diet is limited to clear liquids only after 21'o clock the day before surgery. An enema administered the morning of surgery is recommended. A broad-spectrum antibiotic is administered intravenously 30 min before surgery.

2.4. Patient positioning

The patient is placed in a supine position in slightly Trendelenburg with arms tucked and padded at the sides. Open radical prostatectomy (ORP) was high risk of deep venous thrombosis (DVT). The risk of DVT in LRP is low. However, pelvic lymphadenectomy (PLND) is a risk of DVT in spite of laparoscopic surgery. Sequential compression stocking devices are placed on both legs and activated before surgery. To allow for the access to the rectum, patient's legs are spread apart.

2.5. Surgical technique

2.5.1. Trocars insertion

A right-handed surgeon stands on the left side of the patient. A U-shaped incision is placed on the lower edge of the umbilicus, the subcutaneous fat is divided by the muscle hook, and the rectus abdominal muscle is bluntly peeled off. It is easy to access the space between urachal duct and posterior rectus sheath. Middle finger or index finger is inserted and bluntly peeled off to the arcuate line. A balloon dilator device (PDB balloon, A balloon dilator device (PDB balloon, Coviden Autosuture, Mansfield, MA) is inserted into the preperitoneal space and advanced down to the pubis along the midline. Approximately 500–900 ml of the air is inflated to develop the space of Retzius under direct vision of flexible 5 mm endoscope inserted through the balloon trocar. After removing the balloon trocar, special multi-lumen access device was put in the umbilical incision. Various different devices exist of single-port access, including the GelPort (Applied Medical, Rancho Santa, Margarita, CA), the TriPort (Advanced Surgical Concepts, Bray), and EZ access (Hakko Co. Ltd., Tokyo). Usually, we used EZ access oval type (Hakko Co. Ltd., Tokyo). The cost of EZ access is only $75.7. For example, the price of GelPort is $299.00. A 12 mm and a one 5 mm trocar are inserted into EZ access (to consider cost, reusable trocar is better). Start pneumoperitoneum at 10 mm Hg; 3 mm or 5 mm trocar is inserted into the left lower abdomen (right-handed surgeon) or the left lower abdomen (left-handed surgeon), and next 5 mm trocar is inserted into middle lower abdomen. If necessary, 3 mm or 5 mm port is inserted opposite side of lower abdomen (**Figures 1** and **2**).

2.5.2. Development of Retzius cavity and endo-pelvic fascia incision

The fat in front of prostate is removed from prostate. Anterior surface of prostate is revealed until the deepest of Retzius cavity. Endo-pelvic fascia is incised along both outsides of the prostate gland and the rectal pre-fat is exposed on the dorsal side (**Figure 3**). Preventing inguinal hernia, peritoneum is dissected from seminal duct and vessels.

2.5.3. Dissecting of bladder neck and cutting

The fat outside the bladder prostate boundary is removed as much as possible. The shape of bladder neck is revealed (**Figure 4**) and lateral part of the seminal vesicles is identified before

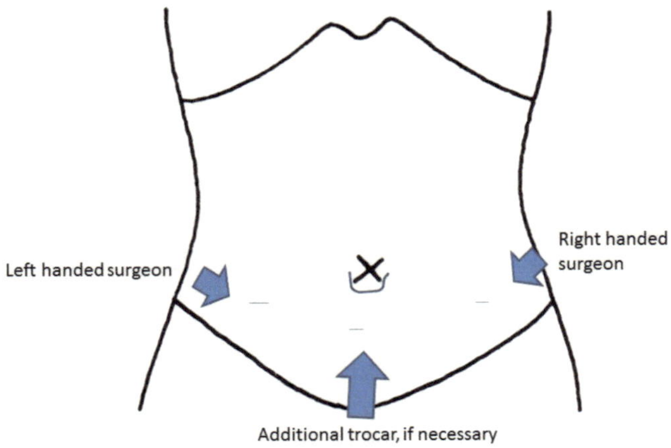

Figure 1. Schema of trocar placement.

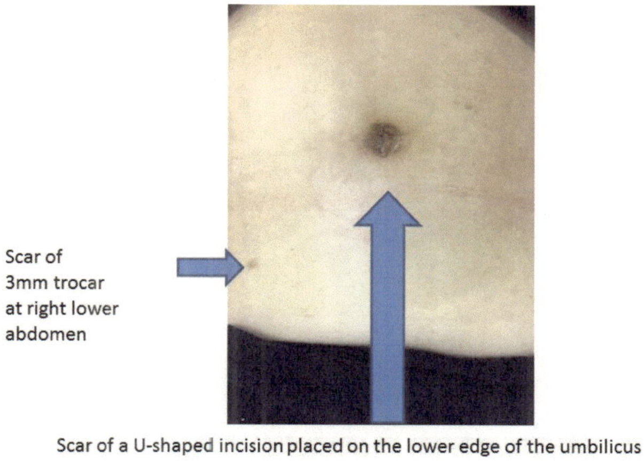

Figure 2. A picture of operative scars after surgery.

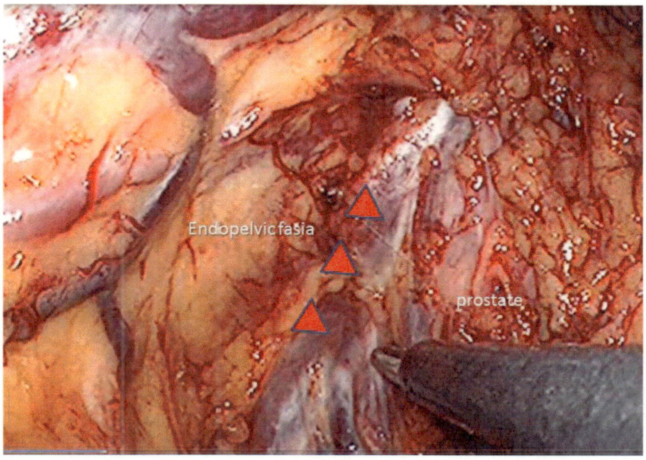

Figure 3. Cutting of endo-pelvic fascia.

bladder neck cutting. Cutting after the internal urethral meatus (**Figure 5**), the vas deferens is identified and cut (**Figure 6**).

2.5.4. Denonvilliers' fascia incision and cutting the prostatic lateral ligament

After dissection of the seminal vesicles from bladder, the seminal vesicles and the vas deferens are lifted up, the Denonvilliers' fascia was incised carefully. The space between the rectum and the prostate is dissected at the midline. The prostatic lateral ligament remaining on the prostate outer side is coagulated and cut (**Figure 7**). It is easy to use a sealing device to proceed without switching the device. To avoid rectal injury, it is important to take care of the line of cutting prostate lateral ligament.

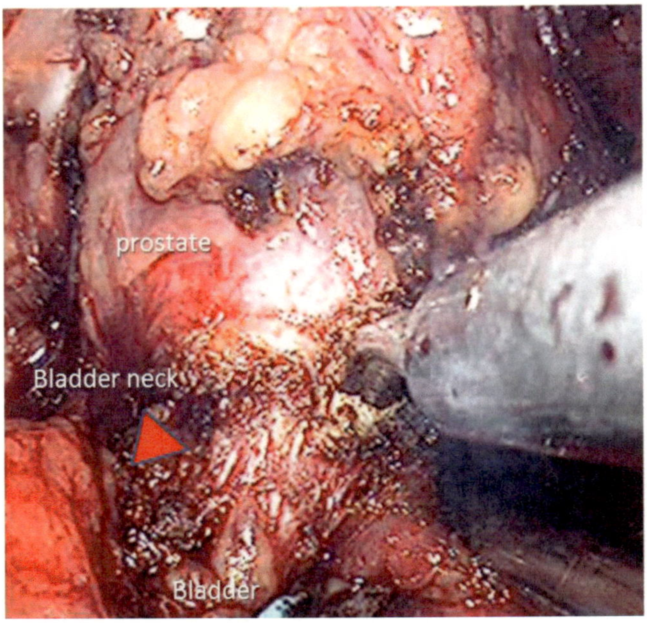

Figure 4. Incision of bladder neck.

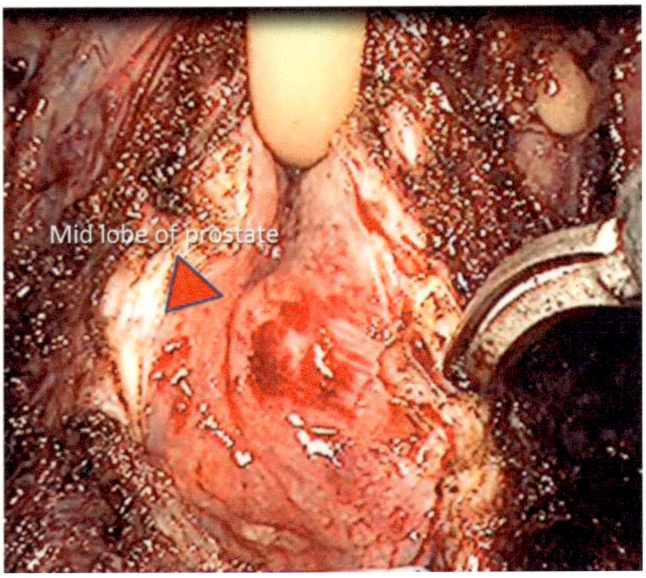

Figure 5. Cutting internal urethral meatus.

When preserving neurovascular bundle, to avoid heat damage, use 5 mm clip and cut with scissors. After cutting the lateral ligaments, the lateral side of urethra is identified.

http://dx.doi.org/10.5772/intechopen.79364

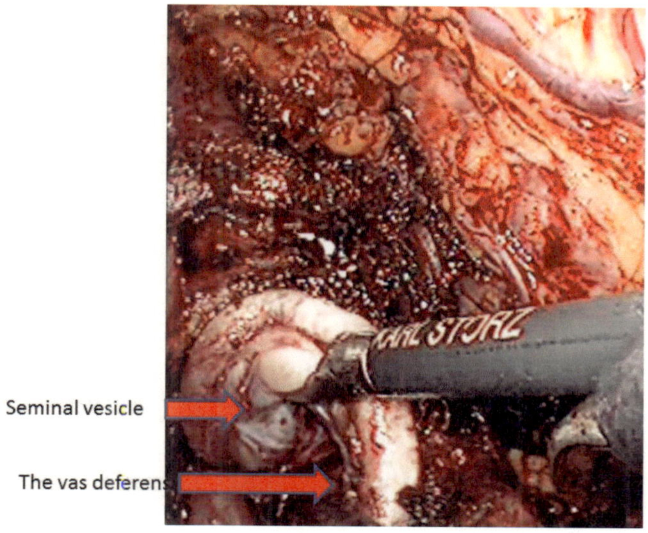

Figure 6. Identify of the vas deferens.

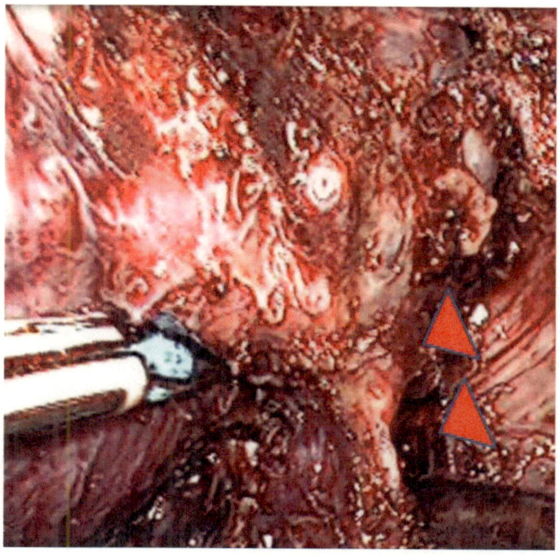

Figure 7. The prostatic lateral ligament.

2.5.5. Bunching and cutting of urethra

Bunching of the DVC with Z suture was done (**Figure 8**). After cutting the DVC proximally, prostate is connecting to the pelvic floor only with the urethra (**Figure 9**). The urethra is cut as much as possible to preserve the urethra confirming the shape of the prostate. The bag is inserted from the umbilicus port, the prostate gland is stored in the bag, and prostate is removed from umbilicus port. If prostate is large, urachal duct is ligated and cut under umbilicus, it is easy to remove prostate. If lymphadenectomy is necessary, lymphadenectomy is done.

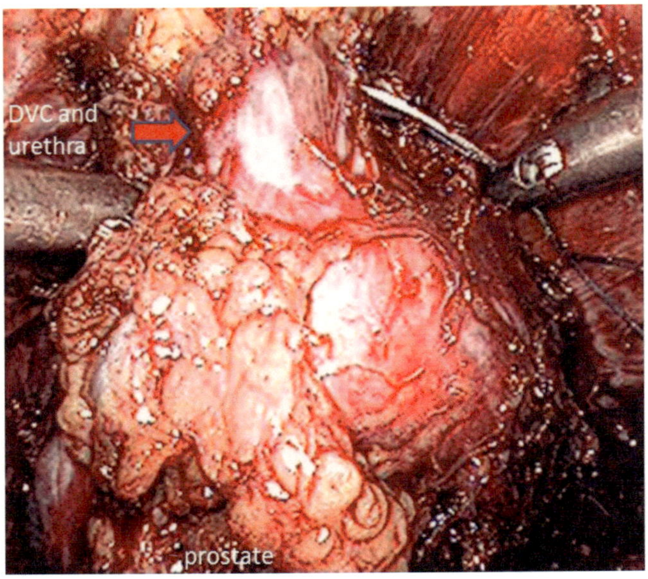

Figure 8. Bunching of DVC.

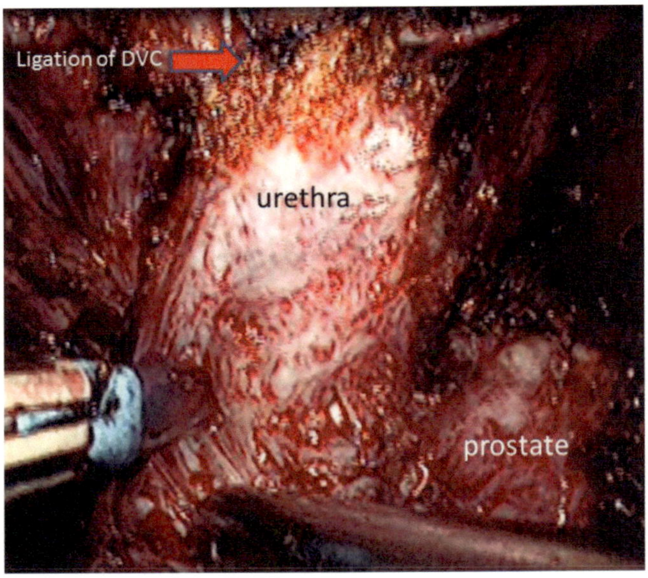

Figure 9. Revealed urethra.

2.5.6. Pelvic lymphadenectomy

Nowadays, lymphadenectomy for diagnosis is not necessary. For several patients with a significant risk for a nodal metastasis, PNLD may be useful for treatment.

Therefore, PLND is recommended in patients with intermediate or high risk.

http://dx.doi.org/10.5772/intechopen.79364

To consider PLND, one more additional trocar is necessary, at middle lower abdomen. To retract the peritoneum, a 5-mm-sized retractor is inserted from the umbilicus port. Seminal duct and vessels are ligated and cut. Cooper's ligaments as a lower edge, adipose tissue is detached along external iliac vein and artery. The outside of LND is along the pelvic floor muscle. Obturator nerve and obturator artery and vein are exposed, and dissection is promoted to the inner iliac artery bifurcation. Next, carefully exfoliate the fat between the obturator vessels and the bladder. A thick lymph duct is treated with a sealing device or 5 mm clip.

2.5.7. *Anastomosis of bladder neck and urethral stump*

The bladder neck and urethral stump are anastomosed using 3-0 monofilament surgical suture at both ends. First, Rocco suturing is performed, after Rocco suturing (**Figure 10**), the rear wall is sutured with a horizontal mattress, and after closing it, the side walls are continuously sewn as they are. Approximately 10 needles are sewn. Place the urinary catheter in the bladder, inject saline, and check for leaks (**Figure 11**). Anterior bladder wall is fixed to pubic bone using 3-0 synthetic absorbable surgical suture.

2.5.8. *Drain insertion*

Incerting the forceps from the left trocar, the tip of the forceps is put the out side of umbilicus port. The end of drain is caught by the forceps and removed from the left trocar. The drain is placed. Usually, drain is removed 2 or 3 days after surgery.

Finally, the wound is closed with buried suture.

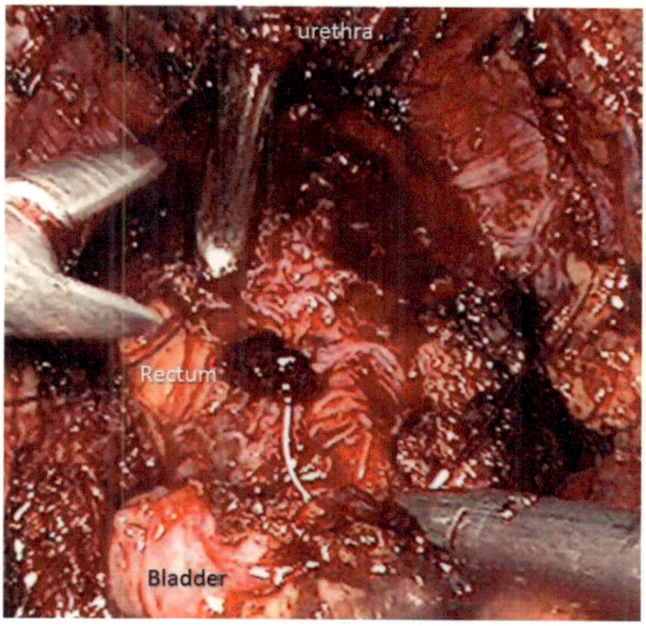

Figure 10. Rocco suturing.

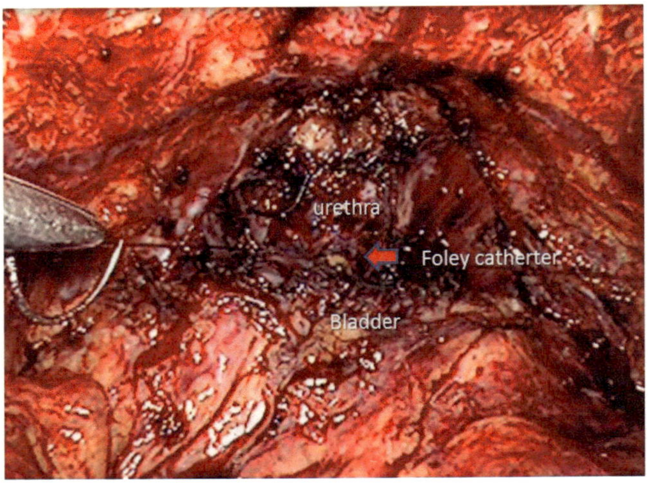

Figure 11. Anastomosis of urethra and bladder.

2.6. Complication

There is no prospective study to compare the efficacy and complication between LRP and reduced port LRP. We think that the quality of reduced port LRP is as same as conventional LRP, because surgical procedure is same. In our experience of LRP, rectal injury occurred in 1% of patients and allogeneic blood transfusion rate was 0% [17].

Rassweiler et al. compared early and late groups of LRP and an open radical prostatectomy group. Mean OR time was 218 min for late laparoscopic surgery and 196 min for open surgery. Transfusion rates were 9.6 and 55.7%, respectively. Complications included rectal injuries (1.4 vs. 1.8%), lymphoceles (0 vs. 6.9%), and anastomotic strictures (4.1 vs. 15.9%, respectively) [18]. Katz et al. reported the incidence of rectal injury is 2% during LRP [19]. Intraoperative recognition of rectal injury is important. When recognizing the rectal injury, multilayer primary closure should be performed before bladder and urethral anastomosis. Filling the water in front of rectum and injection of air into the rectum from anus to check the leaks. When fistula between vesicourethral anastomosis and the rectum, putting temporary artificial anus is necessary. After control of the infection, secondary reconstructive surgery using gracilis muscle flaps between rectum and vesicourethral anastomosis.

Injury of iliac vessels may be occurred during the lateral side trocar placement or along the path of instruments from the lateral side trocar.

The incidence of venous thromboembolism (VTE) of LRP and RALP is very low about 0.5%. However, PLND is the risk of VTE in spite of laparoscopic surgery. Tyritzis et al. reported that the risk of VTE in RALP is 7.52 times when LND is done [20]. The AUA guidelines and EAU guidelines do not recommend the use of prophylactic anticoagulants for LRP and RALP unless patients have known risk of VTE [21, 22]. The use of sequential compression stockings are recommended during the operative and postoperative period.

http://dx.doi.org/10.5772/intechopen.79364

	Reduced port LRP	ORP
No of patients	2	2
Age	67.5 (63-72)	72.5 (72-73)
PSA	5.37 (4.73-6.00)	4.88 (4.51-5.24)
GL score	3+3 / 4+4	3+3 / 4+4
Clinical T	T1c	T1c
Duration of surgery	296 (275-317)	249 (235-258)
Estimated blood loss	225 (100-350)	1602 (1562-1642)
No of using painkiller	1 (0-2)	5 (4-6)
Blood transfusion	None	None
Duration of hospital stay	9	12
Complication	None	None

Table 1. Comparison between reduced port LRP and ORP.

Urinary stricture is rare. In our experience of LRP, the incidence urinary stricture is 2%. Continence rate of 6 months after surgery is 85.9% in our LRP series.

Complications related to patients positioning, such as pressure injury, are rare. To avoid pressure injury, careful padding of vulnerable body parts (the hips, the shoulders, the knees and the calves) is important.

Open conversion is rare, and it usually occurred during a surgeon's early experience with LRP.

From April 2018 to May 2018, four radical prostatectomies were performed. Two cases were reduced port LRP and others were ORP. Two cases done with ORP had a history of lower abdominal open surgery. The results of radical prostatectomy are shown in **Table 1**. The number of the use of painkillers was less in the patients with reduced port LRP than in those of ORP. Estimated blood loss was smaller in those of reduced port LRP than those of ORP. Hospital stay was shorter in reduced port LRP cases.

3. Discussion

The advantages of laparoscopic or robot-assisted radical prostatectomy were significantly decreased blood loss and decreased postoperative pain and shorter convalescence than that of open surgery in spite of similar oncological outcome. However, almost five incisions and one 4–5 cm incision are required. Each incision had a risk of pain, blood loss, internal organs injury, port hernia and infection. According to Chang et al., the number of using analgesic medicine is less in reduced port LRP group than conventional LRP group (3 vs. 19, respectively, p = 0.0318) [23]. In 2008, Kaouk et al. reported first laparoendoscopic single-site radical prostatectomy (LESS-RP), which was performed on four patients with low-risk prostate cancer [24]. All four cases were completed without conversion to a standard laparoscopic approach, and the mean operative time for prostate excision and vesicourethral anastomosis was 3.25 and 1.1 h, respectively. One patient developed a rectourethral fistula that required surgical intervention. The authors concluded that LESS-RP is challenging but feasible. After their report, several studies had also proved its feasibility and safety [23, 25]. However, even with the use of laparoscopic curved or articulating instruments, significant "clashing" with both the camera and other instruments can increase operative times and require significant laparoscopic skills especially for intracorporeal suturing. To overcome the problems, we have focused on reduced port surgery. Akita et al. reported excellent results of 2-port RP comparing with conventional LRP [26]. However, the duration of surgery was longer in 2-port RP than conventional LRP (351.8 ± 72.4 min in 2-port RP and 286.5 ± 63.3 in LRP, P: $p = 0.0019$). Therefore, we performed three or four port RP using 3–5 mm trocar. The procedure is same as conventional LRP and clashing with both the camera and other instruments do not increase. To facilitate smooth instrument manipulation along with adequate visualization during laparoscopy, usually trocars are placed in triangular fashion. In our method, triangulation is kept during operation. We have used conventional straight laparoscopic instruments, such as dissectors, monopolar scissors and needle holders, Ligasure sealing device (Medtronic, Minneapolis, MN), WECK Hem-o-lok® ligation clip and applier (Teleflex Medical, NC), 5 mm flexible scope (Olympus, Tokyo). No other special instruments for LESS. The cost of reduced port LRP (single-port access, four trocars, sealing device) is as same as conventional LRP (five trocars, sealing device).

Hughes et al. reported RALP led to cost savings in the postoperative phase after surgery in a hospital when the cost of the index surgery was excluded. However, Hyldgard et al. reported the use of RALP generates a factor 1.3 additional cost when compared with OP and a factor 1.6 additional cost when compared with LP, on average, based on 12 months follow-up [1]. The median direct cost of RALP is $6752 and that of LRP is $5687. The main difference was in surgical supply costs for each procedure ($2015 for RALP, $725 for LRP) and operation room costs ($2798 for RALP, $2453 for LRP, $1611) [27]. Thus RALP is expensive.

Several authors reported Robot LESS [28–31]. However, it is necessary to buy new da Vinci surgical system for single-port surgery only. It is impossible now because Robot LESS is too expensive surgery however, in the future, Robot LESS become new standard single-port laparoscopic surgery.

4. Conclusion

The procedure of reduced port LRP is the same as conventional LRP. Blood loss is minimal due to tamponade effect of the pneumoperitoneum. The cost of reduced port LRP is cheaper than that of RALP. VTE, rectal injury, and transfusion are rare events. There is no prospective study to compare conventional LRP or RALP with reduced port LRP. Furthermore study is necessary.

http://dx.doi.org/10.5772/intechopen.79364

Acknowledgements

In this manuscript, there is no funding support.

Conflict of interest

We have no conflict of interest.

Author details

Kazuhiro Araki and Yukio Naya*

*Address all correspondence to: nayay@med.teikyo-u.ac.jp

Department of Urology, Teikyo University Chiba Medical Center, Ichihara, Japan

References

[1] Hyldgard V, Laursen KR, Pousen J, et al. Robot-assisted surgery in broader healthcare perspective: A difference-in-difference-based cost analysis of a national prostatectomy cohort. BMJ Open. 2017 Jul 21;**7**(7):e015580

[2] Rabenalt R, Arsov C, Giessing M, et al. Extraperitoneal laparo-endoscopic single-site radical prostatectomy: First experience. World journal of Urology. 2010 Dec;**28**(6):705-708

[3] Herati AS, Atalla MA, Montag S, et al. Laparo-endoscopic single–site radical prostatectomy; Feasubility and technique. Arab journal of Urology. 2011 Mar;**9**(1):73-77

[4] Cáceres F, Cabrera PM, García-Tello A, et al. Safety study of umbilical single-port laparoscopic radical prostatectomy with a new DuoRotate system. European Urology. 2012 Dec;**62**(6):1143-1149

[5] Tugcu V, Ilbey YO, Sonmezay E, et al. Laparoendoscopic single-site versus conventional transperitoneal laparoscopic pyeloplasty: A prospective randomized study. International Journal of Urology. 2013;**20**:1112-1117

[6] Sato F, Nakagawa K, Kawauchi A, et al. Laparoendoscopic single-site surgeries: A multicenter experience of 469 cases in Japan. International Journal of Urology. 2017;**24**:69-74

[7] Hsia M, Ponsky L, Rosenblatt S, Jones JS. Laparoscopic inguinal hernia repair complicates future pelvic oncologic surgery. Annals of Surgery. 2004 Nov;**240**(5):922. author reply 922-3

[8] Cooperberg MR, Downs TM. Carroll PR radical retropubic prostatectomy frustrated by prior laparoscopic mesh herniorrhaphy. Surgery. 2004 Apr;**135**(4):452-453. discussion 454

[9] Katz EE, Patel RV, Sokoloff MH, et al. Bilateral laparoscopic inguinal hernia repair can complicate subsequent radical retropubic prostatectomy. The Journal of Urology. 2002 Feb;**167**(2 Pt 1):637-638

[10] Cook H, Afzal N, Cornaby AJ. Laparoscopic hernia repairs may make subsequent radical retropubic prostatectomy more hazardous. BJU International. 2003 May;**91**(7):729

[11] Brown JA, Dahl DM. Transperitoneal laparoscopic radical prostatectomy in patients after laparoscopic prosthetic mesh inguinal herniorrhaphy. Urology. 2004;**63**:380vii-3380ix

[12] Erdogru T, Teber D, Frede T, et al. The effect of previous transperitoneal laparoscopic inguinal herniorrhaphy on transperitoneal laparoscopic radical prostatectomy. The Journal of Urology. 2006;**173**:769-772

[13] Costas D, Lallas MD, Mark L, et al. Transperitoneal robotic-assisted laparoscopic prostatectomy after prosthetic mesh herniorrhaphy. Journal of the Society of Laparoendoscopic Surgeons. 2009;**13**:142-147

[14] Colombo R, Naspro R, Salonia A, et al. Radical prostatectomy after previous prostate surgery: Clinical and functional outcomes. The Journal of Urology. 2006;**176**(6 Pt 1): 2459-2463

[15] Jaffe J, Stakhovsky O, Cathelineau X, et al. Surgical outcomes for men undergoing laparoscopic radical prostatectomy after transurethral resection of the prostate. The Journal of Urology. 2007;**178**:483-487

[16] Menard J, Taille A, Hoznek A, et al. Laparoscopic radical prostatectomy after transurethral resection of the prostate: Surgical and functional outcomes. Urology. 2008;**72**:593-597

[17] Paul T, Gellhaus PT, Monn F, Leese J, et al. Robot-assisted radical prostatectomy in patients with a history of holmium laser enucleation of the prostate: Feasibility and evaluation of initial outcomes. Journal of Endourology. 2015;**29**(7):764-769

[18] Imamoto T, Goto Y, Utsumi T, et al. Complications, urinary continence, and oncologic outcomes of laparoscopic radical prostatectomy: Single-surgeon experience for the first 100 cases. Prostate Cancer. 2011:7. Article ID 606505

[19] Rassweiler J, Seemann O, Schulze M, Teber D, Hatzinger M, Frede T. Laparoscopic versus open radical prostatectomy: A comparative study at a single institution. Journal of Urology. 2003;**169**(5):1689-1693

[20] Katz R, Borkowski T, Hoznek A, et al. Operative management of rectal injuries during laparoscopic radical prostatectomy. Urology. 2003;**62**(2):310-313

[21] Tyritzis SI, Wallerstedt A, Steineck G, et al. Thromboembolic complications in 3,544 patients undergoing radical prostatectomy with or without lymph node dissection. The Journal of Urology. 2015;**193**:117-125

[22] Violette PD, Cartwright R, Briel M, Tikkinen KA, Guyatt GH. Guideline of guidelines: Thromboprophylaxis for urologic surgery. BJU International. 2016;**118**:351-358

[23] Jiang C, Huang J, Lin T, et al. Extraperitoneal transumbilical laparoendoscopic single-site radical prostatectomy using a homemade single-port device: 20 cases with midterm outcomes. World Journal of Urology. 2014;**32**:829-836

[24] Tikkinen KAO, Cartwright R, Gould MK, et al. EAU Guidelines on Thromboprophylaxis in Urological Surgery. (ISBN: 978-90-79754-91-5) Available from: http://www.uroweb.org/guidelines/

[25] Kaouk JH, Goel RK, Haber GP, et al. Single-port laparoscopic radical prostatectomy. Urology. 2008;**72**:1190-1193

[26] Zhang D-X, Teng J-F, Pan X-W, et al. A matched-pair comparison of single plus one port versus standard extraperitoneal laparoscopic radical prostatectomy by a single urologist. Kaohsiung Journal of Medical Sciences. 2015;**31**:344e350

[27] Akita H, Nakane A, Ando R, et al. Reduced port surgery for prostate cancer is feasible: Comparative study of 2-port laparoendoscopic and conventional 5-port laparoscopic radical prostatectomy. Asian Pacific Journal of Cancer Prevention. 2013;**14**(11):6311-6314

[28] Bolenz C, Gupta A, Hotze T, et al. Cost comparison of robotic, laparoscopic, and open radical prostatectomy for prostate cancer. European Urology. 2010;**57**:453-458

[29] White MA, Haber GP, Autorino R, et al. Robotic laparoendoscopic single-site radical prostatectomy: Technique and early outcomes. European Urology. 2010;**58**:544-550

[30] Kaouk JH, Haber GP, Autorino R, et al. A novel robotic system for single-port urologic surgery: First clinical investigation. European Urology. 2014;**66**:1033-1043

[31] Tugcu V, Simsek A, Evren I, et al. Single plus one port robotic radical prostatectomy (SPORP); initial experience. Archivio Italiano di Urologia, Andrologia. 2017;**89**:3

Section 8

Prostatectomy Recovery and Quality of Life

Preventing Erectile Dysfunction after Radical Prostatectomy: Nerve-Sparing Techniques, Penile Rehabilitation, and Novel Regenerative Therapies

Michael Whalen

Additional information is available at the end of the chapter

http://dx.doi.org/10.5772/intechopen.79398

Abstract

Erectile dysfunction is a known and much-dreaded functional consequence of radical prostatectomy. Dr. Patrick Walsh pioneered the nerve-sparing radical retropubic prostatectomy in the early 1980s, which has mitigated the morbidity of this surgery. Postoperative potency rates range widely from 20 to 80%, however, and depend on myriad factors including age, preoperative potency, and degree of nerve-sparing during surgery. Over the past four decades several developments have continued to offer hope to patients and clinicians alike, including refined understanding of cavernosal nerve neuroanatomy, beneficial modifications in surgical technique, as well as the advent of robotic surgery. Furthermore, multiple pre- and post-operative penile rehabilitation techniques using mechanotherapy and pharmaceuticals have also improved functional recovery. This paper examines erectile dysfunction as a consequence of radical prostatectomy, including the physiology of erections, the pathophysiology of post-operative erectile dysfunction, novel surgical techniques to enhance neurovascular bundle preservation, and penile rehabilitation strategies involving hyperbaric oxygen, neuroprotective pharmaceuticals, dehydrated human amnion-chorion membrane allografts, and mesenchymal stem cell therapy.

Keywords: erectile dysfunction, nerve-traction injury, nerve-sparing radical prostatectomy, penile rehabilitation, amnion-chorion membrane therapy, stem cell therapy

1. Introduction

Erectile dysfunction is a known and much-dreaded functional consequence of surgery for prostate cancer. Although surgeons may cite oncologic control as the paramount component of the

"Trifecta" (i.e. cancer cure, continence, and potency), many patients cite recovery of erectile function as the true measure of treatment success. In the early days of radical prostatectomy, post-operative potency rates were poor, and in fact largely non-existent. With the advent of nerve-sparing anatomic radical retropubic prostatectomy, a surgical approach pioneered by Dr. Patrick Walsh, the prospect of post-operative recovery of potency became not only a possibility but a reality for many men. The myriad factors that influence a patient's likelihood of sexual function recovery after both open and robotic radical prostatectomy have been examined and published in the literature. Also, there has been much investigation into the pathophysiology of iatrogenic erectile dysfunction (i.e. neurapraxia and nerve-traction injury) in the form of in vitro, pre-clinical animal studies and even translational studies with randomized human subjects. Given the pivotal importance of erectile function in a patient's perceived post-operative quality of life, there is much interest in the optimization of perioperative techniques to spare the integrity of the cavernous nerves and to develop efficacious mechanical and pharmacologic penile rehabilitation programs. Such programs employ an increasingly sophisticated arsenal of medical technologies such as pluripotent stem cell therapy, cytokine-rich human amnion-chorion membrane allograft, and even reappropriation of pharmacotherapies traditionally used for other disease states that have been found to have neuroprotective properties. This chapter will examine the evolution in the understanding of erectile dysfunction as a consequence of radical prostatectomy and examine novel strategies for prevention and amelioration of this condition.

2. Physiology of erections

2.1. Anatomy

The central role of smooth muscle dynamics in the corpora cavernosa in the development of erections was first elucidated in the 1980s [1]. Identification of nitric oxide (NO) as the principle neurotransmitter for tumescence and phosphodiesterases for detumescence were also major milestones with well-known pharmacologic ramifications. Anatomically, beneath the Buck's fascia, the corpora cavernosa are surrounded by the two-layered tunica albuginea, a reticulated network of collagen and elastin fibers that provides structural support during tumescence. The outer layer serves to compress the obliquely oriented emissary veins during tumescence that results in the "bottle-neck" effect of slower outflow than inflow that is essential for maintenance of an erection (**Figure 1**) [2]. The penile arterial supply arises from internal pudendal artery, which then gives rise to the common penile artery that branches into the dorsal, cavernous, and bulbourethral arteries. The cavernous arteries are responsible for the engorgement of the corpora cavernosa during tumescence. Accessory pudendal arteries may also be present in up to 4–25% of patients and these arise from the external iliac, obturator, vesical, and femoral arteries. Their preservation has been shown to be important for recovery of erectile function after radical prostatectomy [3, 4].

2.2. Neuroanatomy

The vasomotor tone of the cavernous arteries is regulated by the autonomic cavernous nerves. They are the nerves that are being described during "nerve-sparing" techniques during radical

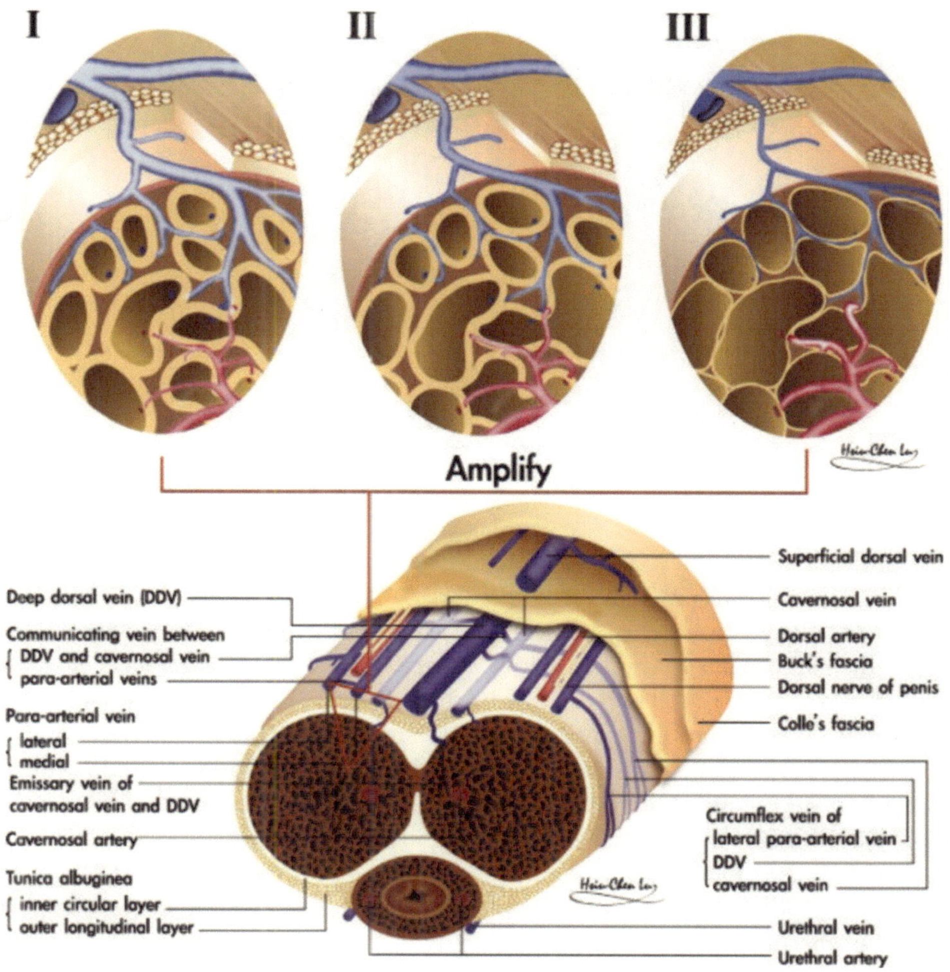

Figure 1. Anatomy of subtunical emissary veins as the basis for tumescence. Reprinted without changes from Molodysky et al. [2] https://creativecommons.org/licenses/by-nc-nd/3.0/.

prostatectomy. These nerves arise as an extension from the parasympathetic pelvic splanchnic nerves that originate from the pelvic plexus (S2–S4) located on either side of the rectum (**Figure 2**). These nerves innervate the endothelium of the cavernous sinuses and release acetylcholine which inhibits adrenergic neurons and stimulates NO release from endothelial cells [5]. NO increases intracellular production of cGMP with resultant decline in intracellular calcium and relaxation of the cavernous smooth muscle. Phosphodiesterase 5 is responsible for the degradation of cGMP and is the target of the well-known medications for erectile dysfunction.

Since Walsh and Donker pioneered the nerve-sparing radical prostatectomy in 1982, there has been much debate about the nature and trajectory of these nerves [6, 7]. These nerves have been found to travel as a latticework of delicate fibers principally along the posterolateral and lateral aspects of the prostate, but with some fibers coursing ventrally as well. Invaluable work in human cadavers by several investigators has elucidated precise position and orientation of these nerves to optimize their preservation during radical prostatectomy.

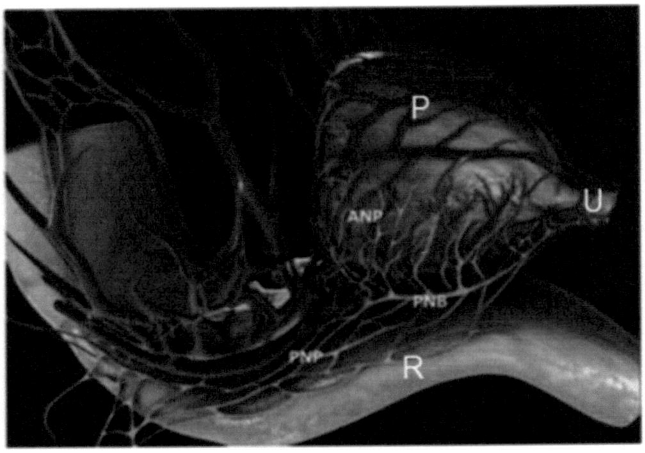

Figure 2. Pelvic plexus and cavernous nerve anatomy. P = prostate; U = urethra; R = rectum; PNP = proximal neurovascular plate; ANP = accessory neurovascular plate; PNB = predominant neurovascular bundle. Reprinted from Tewari et al. [12].

Costello et al. used cadaver models to identify three functional domains of the neurovascular bundle (NVB): the posterior and posterolateral component runs within the Denonvilliers' fascia and the pararectal fascia and innervates the rectum; the lateral component supplies the levator ani, and the cavernosal nerves lie along the posterolateral surface [8, 9]. Furthermore, Lunacek et al. showed that the cavernous nerves are displaced more anteriorly and splay along the lateral aspect of the prostate like a curtain [10]. These findings inspired the "curtain dissection" technique of high anterior release as well as the technique of preserving the lateral prostatic fascia within which the neurovascular bundle travels known as the "Veil of Aphrodite" technique to maximize the number of nerve fibers preserved [10, 11]. Dr. Ashutosh Tewari has conceptualized the neuroanatomy as consisting of a tri-zonal neural architecture, comprised of the proximal neurovascular plate (PNP), predominant neurovascular bundle (PNB), and accessory neural pathways (ANP) [12]. The PNP is synonymous with the pelvic plexus and the PNB is the traditionally described NVB, which is enclosed within the layers of levator fascia and/or lateral pelvic fascia. The nerves are situated in a "hammock-like" distribution rather than a distinct, isolated structure (**Figure 2**).

Further anatomical studies have demonstrated that a significant proportion of the nerves are situated on the anterior surface of the prostate, 21.5–28.5% [13] and 19.9–22.8% (**Figure 3**) [14]. Structural configurations range from round and bundle-like to more widely distributed splay-like [15]. Ganzer et al. employed computerized planimetry software to analyze the topography of the nerves on whole-mount pathologic sections obtained during non-nerve-sparing radical prostatectomy [16]. Total nerve surface area was most concentrated dorsolaterally (74.5–84.1%), but up to 39.9% of nerve surface area was found ventrolaterally. These correspond to the ANPs described by Dr. Tewari's group, who found them in 41% of the cadavers [12]. It is possible that all of these nerves are not responsible for erections. Subsequent studies in electrophysiologic stimulation have shown cavernosal pressure responses with stimulation at all positions of the midprostate between the 1:00 and 5:00 positions for all patients, suggesting their role in potency [17]. The precision vs. degree of electrical spread of such electrical stimulation may represent a limitation of this testing. Conversely, Costello et al. reported that

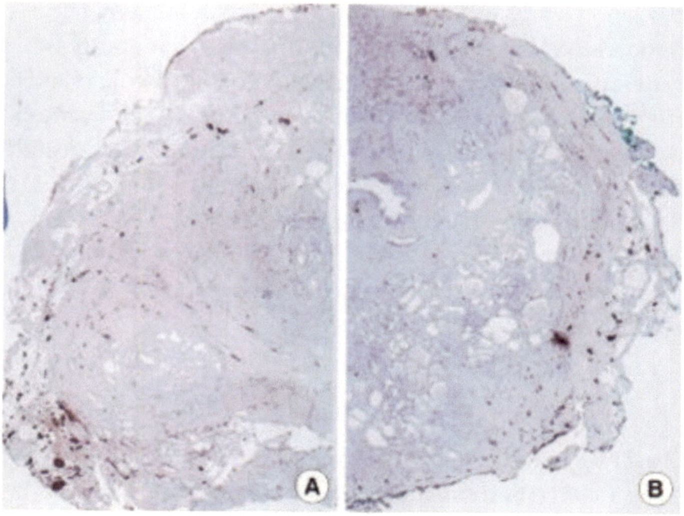

Figure 3. Whole-mount anatomy of neurovascular bundle (NVB) topography on the prostate. A. NVB concentrated at posterolateral aspect of prostate (S-100 stain) B. NVB are more widely distributed to ventral aspect of prostate (S-100 stain). Reprinted from Lee et al. [14].

significantly parasympathetic nerve fibers only account for 4–6.8% of nerves on the anterolateral aspect of the prostate [18]. These findings were corroborated by Ganzer et al., who used immunohistochemistry to distinguish between parasympathetic and sympathetic nerves. They reported that only 14.6% of the parasympathetic nerves resided above a horizontal line drawn at the prostate base and only 1.5% above a horizontal line at the apex [19].

How these anatomical findings impact the functional outcomes of the various nerve-sparing approaches described below, some of which advocate for high anterior release of the prostatic fascia, is interesting to consider (see Section 5.2).

3. Pathophysiology of post-prostatectomy erectile dysfunction

There are several acute and chronic factors that contribute to decline in erectile function after surgery for prostate cancer. These factors may be classified as vasculogenic, neurogenic, and even psychological. The burden of cancer diagnosis, treatment, and need for long-term PSA monitoring, along with recovery from surgery, implications on self-image, awareness of mortality, and perceived or actual reduction in penile length represent a constellation of psychosocial factors that may contribute to ED.

The role of accessory pudendal arteries in vasculogenic erectile function has been described above. Chen et al. has also implicated the veins that travel longitudinally within the layers of the tunica albuginea. His group have reported that ligation of the DVC during prostatectomy results in dilatation of these veins which results in veno-occlusive dysfunction [20].

The vascular sequelae of radical prostatectomy were investigated by Mulhall et al., who reported cavernosometry and/or penile duplex ultrasonography [21]. They found arterial insufficiency in 59% and venous leakage in 26% of men after bilateral nerve-sparing RRP who had excellent pre-operative erectile function. Normal vascular status was found in 35% of men. Return to penetrative function was correlated with the vascular status, with 47% return if normal status, 31% in arteriogenic insufficiency, and only 9% with veno-occlusive dysfunction at 12 months. They also reported that the longer the duration of erectile dysfunction, the higher the risk of venous leakage. Zelefsky et al. reported venous leakage in 52%, arterial insufficiency in 32%, and neurogenic dysfunction in 12% [22]. Montorsi et al. found a higher proportion of patients with veno-occlusive disease in their randomized study of intracavernous alprostadil after open RP: 67% veno-occlusive dysfunction, 17% arterial insufficiency, 17% normal vascular dynamics [23].

3.1. Neurapraxia

The neurogenic basis for erectile dysfunction implicates the cavernous nerve architecture. Preservation of these architectural substrates may not be sufficient alone to engender recovery of post-operative function, as suggested by the well-documented latency period between surgery and functional recovery. This latency ranges from 6–24 months and has been suggested to be the result of nerve-traction injury from the physical manipulation/handling during surgery and resultant neurapraxia and axonotmesis [1, 24, 25].

Intraoperative manipulation and injury to the cavernosal nerves results in hemodynamic and histologic changes within the penis, which manifest clinically as erectile dysfunction. This injury may result from mechanical or thermal sources. Iatrogenic traction on the delicate neurovascular tissue can cause-stretch induced nerve injury and resulting dysfunction. Neuropathies may be classified into three histologic groups: neurapraxia, axonotmesis, and neurotmesis. Neurapraxia is the least severe and is characterized intact neural structural elements, but there may be ischemia and/or demyelination which leads to signal conduction block. Functional deficits in peripheral nerves manifest as motor, proprioceptive, and soft touch deficiencies, but these usually resolve in a few weeks (up to 12 weeks) [26]. The next level of injury is axonotmesis in which axons and their myelin sheaths over long segments of nerve are disrupted, while supporting structures such as the endoneurium are left intact [27]. There is consequent Wallerian degeneration distal to the level of injury and proximal axonal degeneration to the next node of Ranvier. Since the endoneurial tubes remain intact, recovery should be complete after a matter of several months but may not be complete. Frank transection of the nerve is termed neurotmesis, in which the endoneurial tubes and connective tissue components are disrupted. Intraneural fibrosis develops and impairs axonal regeneration and thus inhibits nerve functional recovery. Peripheral nerve regeneration is mediated by multiple factors including neurotrophic factors, extracellular matrix, and intact cellular components of the nervous system (i.e. endoneurium) [28]. Tissue trauma from surgery also generates an inflammatory response and oxidative stress around the degenerating axons with results in chromatolysis (degradation of the protein synthesizing infrastructure of the neuronal cell body) [29].

Nerve injury may have a vasculogenic etiology as well. Nerve ischemia may be a result of direct compression injury or stretch ("traction") injury, which produces a reduction in cross-sectional area and resultant compression of the vasculature [27]. Traction disrupts and occludes small-sized arteries traveling with the nerves (vasa nervorum) which supply pelvic tissues as well as the nerves themselves. Biochemically within the cavernosal smooth muscle cells, hypoxia induces production of superoxide which initiates oxidative reactions and attacks surrounding molecules to produce more free radicals. Oxygen free radicals in the setting of a nitric-oxide containing environment tends to combine to form peroxynitrite (O=NOO-) which is highly neurotoxic. Exposure of nerves to this compound leads to rapid excitation, excitotoxicity, and degeneration in the acute setting. Nitric oxide bioavailability is thereby reduced in this setting, which further impacts penile smooth muscle relaxation and exacerbates the hypoxic conditions.

3.2. Thermal injury

The importance of athermal dissection has been reinforced as classic teaching during nerve-sparing radical prostatectomy. The precise functional deficits induced by monopolar or bipolar cautery has been investigated in a canine model [30]. A total of 12 dogs were divided into four groups of neurovascular bundle dissection: Group 1, suture ligatures; Group 2, monopolar electrocautery; Group 3, bipolar electrocautery; Group 4, ultrasonic shears. Peak intracavernous pressures in response to distal cavernous nerve stimulation immediately post-op and at 2 weeks showed an attenuated response compared to controls (74–91% decrease and 93–96% decrease, respectively). In the dogs where electrocautery was employed, there was in fact almost no rise in the intracavernous pressure in response to stimulation. The findings in this study were presented in the context of having spared the contralateral neurovascular bundle from any dissection. Their results may have been even more dramatic if thermal energy had been used bilaterally. The follow-up was also admittedly short in this series at 2 weeks post-op only. Much longer durations at 6-, 12-, and even 24 months would be helpful to determine the long-term impact of thermal energy on recovery of potency (see Section 5.6).

This very objective was explored in humans after robotic prostatectomy, demonstrating delayed recovery after 12–18 months, but with 68% of bilateral nerve-sparing patient ultimately recovering function at 24 months [31] (see Section 5.3).

3.3. Chronic cavernosal tissue changes

In the chronic phase of injury, the persistent loss of nerve signal conduction results in loss of spontaneous nocturnal erections and relative cavernosal ischemia. The pathophysiologic consequence is cavernosal smooth muscle apoptosis, upregulation of TGF-beta and collagen deposition within the corpora [32–35]. Cavernous neurotomy studies in rats have demonstrated that corporal smooth muscle apoptosis begins 1 day after injury and peaks within the first week [34]. This fibrotic reaction impairs full expansion of the venous sinuses within the tunica and failure to adequately compress the emissary veins against the tunica. The result is "veno-occlusive dysfunction" in which the venous outflow occurs with the same velocity as arterial inflow. In this setting, tumescence is unable to be achieved or maintained. Furthermore, there is anatomical loss of penile length and girth as a result of the cavernosal smooth muscle fibrosis.

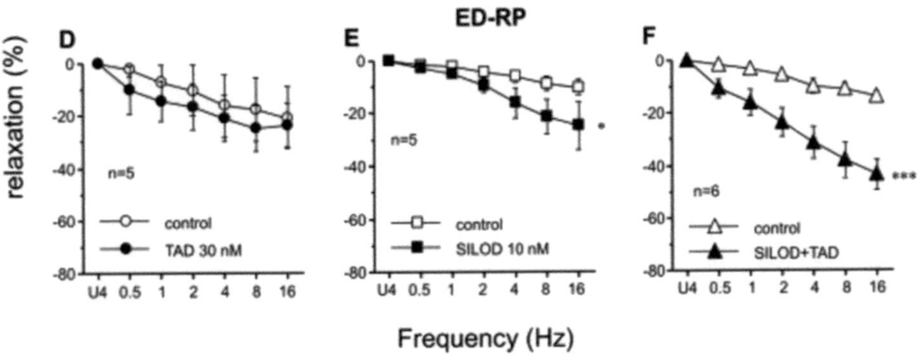

Figure 4. Effects of tadalafil, silodosin, or their combination on neurogenic relaxations induced by electrical field stimulation in human corpus cavernosum strips obtained from patients with erectile dysfunction after RP (ED-RP). *P < 0.05, *** P < 0.001. Reprinted from Martinez-Salamanca et al. [41].

3.4. Sympathetic disinhibition

Erectile function is not only the result of parasympathetic input, but a dynamic interplay between enhanced parasympathetic and inhibited sympathetic function. The role of adrenergic, sympathetic signals in ejaculation and detumescence have been well-established [36]. The adrenergic system essentially inhibits tumescence via the release of presynaptic norepinephrine (NE) that binds to postsynaptic α1- and α2-adrenergic receptors that induce penile arterial and cavernosal smooth muscle contraction. Also, the activation of presynaptic adrenergic receptors on the parasympathetic nerves inhibits release of NO [37]. The α1 receptor subtype is predominant in human erectile tissue, and furthermore α1A and α1D are more common than α1B in humans [38, 39]. Neurogenic contractile responses have been shown to be increased in the corpus cavernosum from rats after cavernous nerve injury and in cavernosal tissues from men with post-prostatectomy ED [40].

Recent animal studies have elucidated the role of adrenergic function on the contractile dynamics of cavernosal smooth muscle [41]. After bilateral crush injury to the cavernosal nerves rats were administered phentolamine (non-selective alpha-blocker), silodosin (α1A-selective alpha-blocker), or tap water only for 4 weeks and intracavernosal pressure (ICP) was monitored after (1) electrical stimulation of the cavernosal nerve proximal to the region of injury and (2) IV administration of tadalafil (phosphodiesterase 5 inhibitor). A significantly greater increase in ICP was observed for the silodosin group compared to the phentolamine or tap water groups after both electrical stimulation alone and co-administration with IV tadalafil. These findings suggest therapeutic benefit to alpha blockade for recovery of erectile function after RP. The authors translated their experiments to humans by obtaining strips of cavernosal smooth muscle at the time of inflatable penile prosthesis insertion. The response to electrical stimulation ex-vivo was enhanced by pretreatment of the muscle strips with both silodosin and tadalafil compared to tadalafil alone (**Figure 4**) [41].

4. Epidemiology of erectile dysfunction

The prevalence of erectile dysfunction in the general population has been reported by two large surveys: the Massachusetts Male Aging Study (MMAS) and the National Health and

Social Life Survey (NHSLS). According to the MMAS the rate of complete, moderate, and mild ED for the study of n = 1709 community-dwelling men in their 40–70 seconds was 5.1–15, 17–34, and 17%, respectively [42]. The NHSLS examined n = 1410 community-dwelling men and women in 1992 and reported rates of ED by age: 7%, 18–29 years; 9% 30–39 years; 11% 40–49 years; 18%, 50–59 years [43]. The definition of ED in this study was not quantified with validated questionnaires. International studies have reported rates of 20–40% for men 60–69 years [44]. ED is therefore an age-dependent disease. Other established risk factors include diabetes mellitus, hypertension, hyperlipidemia, psychiatric/psychologic disorders, history of pelvic trauma, chronic disease states (i.e. hypogonadism, thyroid disease, chronic kidney disease), and socio-demographic status.

There are multiple validated questionnaires to accurately assess various aspects of a patient's baseline sexual function. These questionnaires are integral in the patient workup as both a quantifiable measure of their function and a method of realistic prognostication of their likelihood of meaningful recovery. These elements comprise an important aspect of patient preoperative counseling and informed consent. The International Index of Erectile Function (IIEF) consists of 15 items and five domains and was developed by an international panel of experts for uses in determining treatment efficacy in clinical trials [45, 46]. Given its high sensitivity for detecting clinically significant treatment effects, it is regarded as the gold standard treatment outcome measure. Administration of this long questionnaire is somewhat cumbersome in a routine clinic setting, however. The National Institutes of Health's Consensus Panel on ED lead the development of an abridged five-item version of the IIEF, called the IIEF-5 or the Sexual Health Inventory for Men (SHIM). The SHIM is a powerful grading system and easily-administered patient reported tool [47]. It has high sensitivity and specificity and has been shown to be more reliable than a single item self-assessment of severity of ED [48]. Each question is rated on a Likert scale from 1 to 5, and consists of: "Over the past 6 months":

1. How do you rate your confidence that you could get and keep an erection?

2. When you had erections with sexual stimulation, how often were your erections hard enough for penetration (entering your partner)?

3. During sexual intercourse, how often were you able to maintain your erection after you had penetrated (entered) your partner?

4. During sexual intercourse, how difficult was it to maintain your erection to completion of intercourse?

5. When you attempted sexual intercourse, how often was it satisfactory for you?

Based on response to the questions, men may be categorized into one of five grades of ED severity: no ED (SHIM 22–25), mild (17–21), mild to moderate (12–16), moderate (8–11), severe (1–7). Although there have been multiple other questionnaires published—the Quality of Erection Questionnaire, the Erectile Dysfunction Inventory of Treatment Satisfaction (EDITS), the Self-Esteem and Relationship questionnaire (SEAR); the Erection Hardness Score (EHS), the Sexual Experience Questionnaire—the IIEF and SHIM are the most widely employed, and have indeed been translated into over 30 languages [49, 50]. Another popular health-related quality of life (HRQoL) questionnaire specific to prostatectomy patients is the

Expanded Prostate Cancer Index Composite (EPIC), which examines urinary, bowel, sexual, and hormonal domains [51]. Some of these validated instruments have been used to measure outcomes in the randomized penile rehabilitation studies (see below).

Studies of ED prevalence among men prior to undergoing radical prostatectomy report potency rates ranging from 43 to 84%; the 43% value was obtained through interrogation with the IIEF [52–54]. The landmark prospective Prostate Cancer Outcomes Study (PCOS) included n = 3533 men from the Surveillance, Epidemiology and End Results (SEER) cancer registries diagnosed with prostate cancer in 1994–1995. A total of n = 1288 men who underwent radical prostatectomy had completed a baseline questionnaire were included. Baseline erections firm enough for intercourse was 81%, with 49% reporting a least "little/some" difficulty in maintaining erections [52, 53]. A limitation of these figures, however, is the fact the FDA approval of sildenafil only occurred in 1998 and "baseline" function was assessed through post-hoc recall within 6 months after treatment in 90% of patients, thereby introducing recall bias.

4.1. Incidence of erectile dysfunction after radical prostatectomy

Recovery rates after bilateral nerve-sparing open RRP ranges from 31 to 86% of sexually active men with organ-confined disease [55]. The recovery rates for unilateral nerve-sparing range from 13 to 56%, and for non-nerve sparing 0–17% [56–60]. The CaPSURE database of community-based Urology practices has reported that only 20% of men return to preoperative baseline potency at 12 months after RP [61]. The metric for assessment has an impact on the incidence of ED, and the use of validated questionnaires such as the IIEF tends to expose higher incidence of ED [55]. The long-term outcomes of the PCOS study demonstrated [53] worse erectile function in men after RP compared to radiation therapy at the 2- and 5-year evaluation time points, odds ratio 3.46 and 1.96, respectively. There was no significant difference at the 15-year follow-up time point, however. Defining sexual function as "erections in sufficient for intercourse" produced absolute rates of ED at 2, 5, and 15 years of 78.8, 75.7, and 87%, respectively (**Figure 5**). Of note, only 14.5% of men underwent bilateral nerve-sparing surgery in this series.. Among men who had bilateral nerve-sparing, 5-year erectile function firm enough for intercourse was reported in 40% of men vs. 23% and 23% for unilateral nerve-sparing and no nerve-sparing, respectively. Age was a significant predictor on multivariable analysis. Some limitations were the late approval of sildenafil in 1998 and the fact that RP was performed in an open manner, which limits applications to modern series. During the 3 years prior to the 5 year evaluation, only 43% of men had tried sildenafil.

Contemporary robotic prostatectomy series demonstrate 12 month potency rates ranging from 70 to 80% [62]. A systematic review and meta-analysis of 15 case series totaling n = 3491 patients reported 12- and 24-month potency rates ranging from 54–90% to 63–94%, respectively [63]. Among patients who had bilateral nerve-sparing, 12- and 24-month potency rates were 74 and 82% respectively. There may be a learning-curve effect with the robotic prostatectomy outcomes as well. The impact of surgeon experience/learning has been reported, but did not demonstrate statistical significance for potency rates between cases 1–300, 301–500, and 501–700 (61, 63, 65%, respectively) [64].

Outcomes stratified by specific nerve-sparing approach are presented below (see Section 5.3 below).

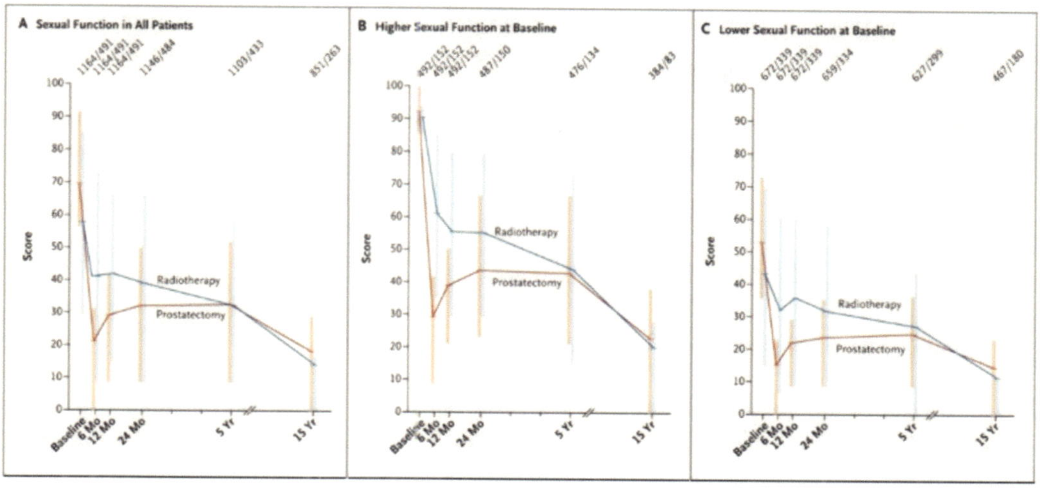

Figure 5. Sexual function over 15 years after treatment for prostate cancer. A. In all patients. B. Higher sexual function with International Index of Erectile Function (IIEF) score > or = 80; C. Lower sexual function, IIEF < 80. Numbers represent total of patients in radical prostatectomy (RP) group/radiation group. Reprinted from Resnick et al. [53].

4.2. Prognostic factors for recovery of erectile function post-prostatectomy

Factors for successful recovery of erectile function have been examined for patients after both open radical retropubic prostatectomy (RRP) and robotic prostatectomy in the modern era. A systematic review post-RRP identified age <60 years, completeness of nerve-sparing, and pre-operative sexual function [55]. Indeed, in the PCOS study a significantly higher proportion of men <60 years reported satisfactory response to sildenafil compared to older men ($p = 0.01$) [52]. The systematic review of robotic prostatectomy by Ficarra et al. cited age, baseline potency status, comorbidities index, and extent of nerve-sparing as predictors of postoperative recovery of potency [63]. There may be a learning-curve effect with the robotic prostatectomy outcomes as well. As discussed below, since nerve-sparing may be performed in an incremental manner rather than an "all-or-none" phenomenon, grade of nerve sparing has shown an influence on recovery [12, 65, 66] (see **Techniques of Nerve Sparing** below).

The impact of surgeon experience/learning has been reported [67], but did not demonstrate statistical significance for potency rates between cases 1–300, 301–500, and 501–700 (61, 63, 65%, respectively) [64]. As mentioned previously, lack of electrocautery during neurovascular bundle dissection portends earlier recovery of erectile function [31]. While other factors have been cited, the previous predictors are the most consistent throughout the medical literature.

Post-operative potency rates may be influenced by the time point of assessment. Studies typically report 12 and 24 month outcomes as the longest follow-up. Although recovery typically occurs within the first 2 years after surgery, delayed recovery is also possible. A series of $n = 1003$ men who underwent either open or robotic RP between 2007 and 2013 reported on the achievement of "good erectile function" as defined by IIEF-6 score ≥ 22 [68]. Among men with poor function at 12 months, the probability of recovering erectile function at 24, 36, and 48 months was 22, 32, and 40% on Kaplan–Meier analysis. The 12-month functional score and patient age were the only significant predictors of delayed recovery on multivariable analysis.

Also, very interestingly, the degree of nerve-sparing was not a predictor of delayed recovery; perhaps nerve-sparing only impacts early recovery at the 12-month time point. Surgical modality (open vs. robotic) was not explored. Similar findings of delayed recovery have been published in other reports [69, 70]. Such findings may be tempered by the gradual decline in erectile function after year 5 observed in the Prostate Cancer Outcomes Study [52].

5. Methods to improve nerve-sparing

5.1. Preoperative planning with multi-parametric MRI

Multiparametric magnetic resonance imaging (mpMRI) has gained widespread use in the workup of elevated PSA and diagnosis of prostate cancer via MRI-transrectal ultrasound (TRUS) targeted fusion biopsy. This technique has been shown to increase the detection rate of high-grade (i.e. Gleason 4 + 3 = 7) prostate cancer by 30% and result in lower detection of low grade prostate cancers by 17% [71]. The recently published PROMIS trial evaluated the performance of mpMRI to the reference standard template prostate mapping (TPM) biopsy and reported superior sensitivity for mpMRI compared to TRUS biopsy (93% vs. 48%, $p < 0.001$) and negative predictive value (89% vs. 74%, $p < 0.001$), allowing 24% with negative MRI to safely avoid having to undergo biopsy [72].

The utility of MRI may be applied to the domain of pre-surgical planning as well. The aggressiveness of nerve-sparing is not solely based on surgeon experience, but also on the anatomical location of the tumor and the presence of locally advanced (i.e. pT3a-b) disease that may be invading the neurovascular bundle. In the setting of pT3 disease (i.e. extraprostatic extension (EPE) and seminal vesicle invasion (SVI)), aggressive nerve sparing may result in a positive surgical margin (PSM), which has been associated with increased rates of biochemical recurrence, systemic metastasis, and prostate cancer-specific mortality post-prostatectomy, especially for high grade disease (i.e. Gleason Score 8–10) [73]. Even with careful adherence to surgical technique and the use of intraoperative frozen section analysis, microscopic positive margins may be imperceptible during surgery. A meta-analysis of 75 studies comprising 9796 patients who underwent mpMRI between 2000 and 2015 demonstrated high specificity for the detection of EPE (90%) and SVI (95%) [74]. However, sensitivity for these endpoints in the best performing series was 71–73%. Therefore, mpMRI may be limited in detecting microscopic EPE and SVI, which surely impacts the safety of nerve-sparing, especially in high risk patients.

Despite these limitations, there is level one evidence published by a single center in Norway suggesting that preoperative mpMRI does indeed reduce the rate of positive surgical margins at robotic radical prostatectomy and influences the rate of nerve-sparing in patients who otherwise might not have been considered for a nerve-sparing approach [75]. Among the $n = 438$ men randomized in this study to preoperative MRI vs. no MRI, sensitivity and specificity for detection of pT3 disease was 73 and 65%, respectively. The mpMRI information altered surgical approach in 27% of patients. Bilateral nerve sparing was performed 6.7% less frequently in the mpMRI group. The positive margin rate was reduced in the mpMRI group for cT1c patients (16% vs. 27%, $p = 0.035$). Among the patients found to have pT3 disease, 89% of them had only unilateral nerve sparing or no nerve sparing. This group did not have improvement in positive margin rate with the mpMRI, however. Perhaps, even wider excision is required to render these patients free of positive margins, which has implications for post-operative potency. Further study is surely needed to clarify the role of mpMRI for pre-surgical planning.

5.2. Intraoperative nerve-sparing techniques

Refined understanding of the neuroanatomy of the cavernous nerves informs the surgical approach to and completeness of nerve-sparing. The endopelvic fascia is a multilayered sheath that encloses and buttresses the prostate and bladder and attaches these organs to the pubic bone via the puboprostatic ligaments. This fascia fuses as the arcus tendineus fascia pelvis just lateral to these organs. The fascial investments of the prostate may be further divided into the prostatic "capsule," periprostatic veins with their fascia, the lateral pelvic fascia (prostatic fascia), levator fascia, and levator ani muscles (**Figure 6**) [76]. Lepor and Walsh described nerve sparing in 1983, with the approach beginning at the prostate apex and proceeding in a retrograde fashion toward the prostatic vascular pedicle [6, 7]. In the modern era of minimally invasive and robotic techniques, the nerve-sparing is usually performed in an antegrade manner after first controlling the prostatic vascular pedicle. Initial experiences with robotic prostatectomy employed monopolar or bipolar electrocautery to control the pedicle until the detrimental role of thermal injury was fully appreciated.

Classical approaches to nerve-sparing have been described as "interfascial" vs. "intrafascial" techniques, as well as the "extra-fascial" approach when nerve-sparing is not performed (**Figure 7**). Interfascial dissection follows the plane lateral to the prostatic fascia, which may render the NVB prone to partial resection. The intrafascial technique follows the plane directly on the prostatic capsule, medial to the prostatic fascia and anterior to the Denonvilliers' fascia, especially at the 5:00 and 7:00 positions. Dissection is typically performed with both blunt and sharp dissection in an athermal manner to reduce transmission of heat and electricity to the proximal NVB.

Refinements in the understanding of the neuroanatomy have resulted in more sophisticated classifications of nerve-sparing. An important concept is the ability to perform incremental nerve sparing, not just as an "all-or-none" phenomenon. It has been suggested that optical magnification and the extended degree of freedom afforded by robotic surgery facilitates

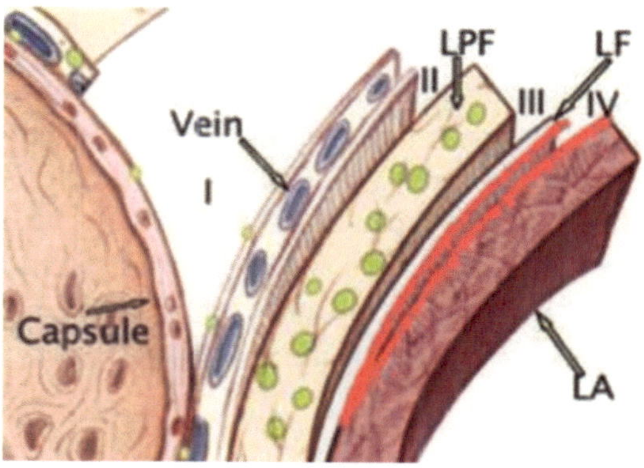

Figure 6. Planes for dissection of nerve-sparing based on prostatic fascial layers. LPF = lateral pelvic fascia (prostatic fascia); LF = levator fascia; LA = levator ani. Reprinted from Tewari et al. [76].

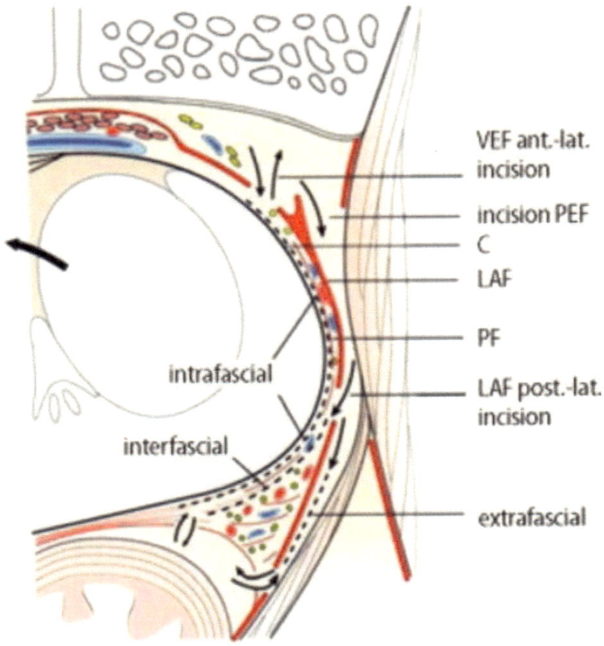

Figure 7. Intrafascial, Interfascial, Extrafascial dissection planes as the basis for nerve-sparing. VEF ant.-lat. = visceral endopelvic fascia anterior-lateral; PEF = parietal endopelvic fascia; C = capsule of prostate; LAF post.-lat. = levator ani fascia posterior-lateral; PF = prostatic fascia. Reprinted from Walz et al. [9].

development of dissection planes within the NVB itself to perform partial nerve sparing in the setting of concern for pT3 disease [12, 77]. This concept is illustrated in **Figure 6**. Dr. Tewari's series of n = 2317 patients was published in 2011 [76]. This approach relies on a risk-stratified approach to the "neural-hammock" as defined by the periprostatic veins and based on preoperative risk stratification based on Gleason score, PSA, digital rectal examination (DRE) findings, cancer volume, and mpMRI findings. The plane of dissection follows one of the grades illustrated in **Figure 6**. A similar grading system based on periprostatic arterial anatomy, rather than venous anatomy, has been proposed by Schatloff et al. (**Figure 8**). In their smaller series of n = 132 patients, they cite a landmark periprostatic artery to define grades as: 1, no nerve sparing; 2, <50% nerve-sparing; 3, 50% nerve sparing; 4, 75% nerve-sparing; 5, ≥95% nerve sparing [78]. The Menon et al. series reported on n = 2652 patients for whom nerve-sparing was initiated by incising the prostatic fascia anteriorly, termed "high anterior release" or the "Veil of Aphrodite" technique (**Figure 9**) [79]. The authors originally reported the development of a plane between the prostatic capsule and prostatic fascia cranially at the base of the seminal vesicles. This plane is propagated deep to the periprostatic venous sinuses with careful blunt and sharp dissection. For patients with significant periprostatic fibrosis after biopsy that impairs development of this plane, the authors recommend initiation of the dissection at the 2:00 or 10:00 position [79].

5.3. Outcomes of nerve-sparing techniques

Comparison of potency rates after the various surgical techniques is not straightforward, as there may be differences in patient demographics such as age and baseline potency,

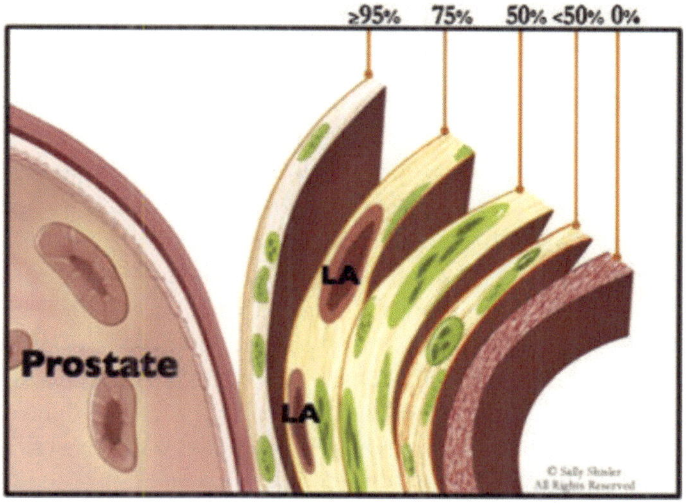

Figure 8. Grades of nerve-sparing based on anatomic landmark of periprostatic artery. LA = landmark artery. Reprinted from Schatloff et al. [78].

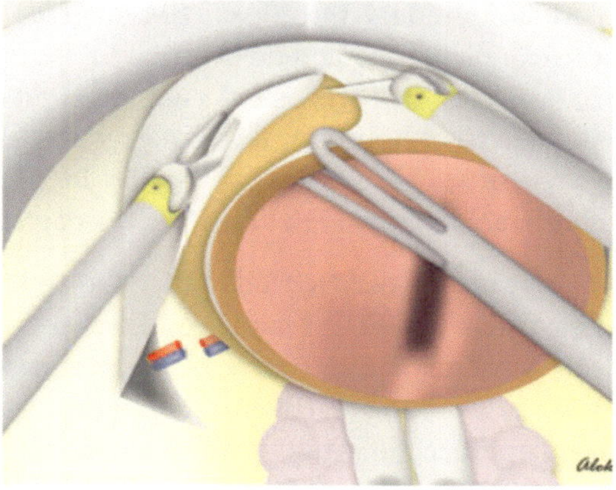

Figure 9. Plane of dissection for Veil of Aphrodite nerve-sparing technique. Reprinted from Menon et al. [79].

as well as tumor characteristics such as stage and grade that may influence the ability to perform bilateral nerve-sparing. Furthermore, based on the aforementioned variations in neuroanatomy among different patients, perfect execution of a given surgical technique may not be enough to accommodate a particular patient's anatomy, resulting in the variability of erectile function recovery. Definitions of potency also vary, with some studies reporting percentage return at a given time point or "return to baseline." The most robust series employ the validated questionnaires (IIEF, SHIM, EPIC), but precise cut-offs for restoration of function may vary. To add the possibility of subjective satisfaction beyond the numbers of the questionnaires, some studies also define potency as "erections suitable for intercourse" that are "satisfactory."

In the setting of these limitations, a recent systematic review and meta-analysis of six studies (only one randomized and three prospective; 4/6 minimally invasive approach) of n = 1663 patients reported improved erectile function at 6 months (RR 1.49) and 12 months (RR 1.40) for intrafascial vs. interfascial nerve-sparing.

Erectile function is not the only component of the Trifecta directly affected by nerve-sparing. Oncologic control with regard to the presence of positive surgical margins is also very important. Given the increased rates of biochemical recurrence and possibility of increased rates of metastasis and prostate-cancer specific mortality associated with the presence of a positive surgical margin, nerve-sparing outcomes must be understood within the context of margin status. Overall, the rates of PSM are around 15%, with rates ranging from 6 to 38% and influenced by pathologic stage, grade, and D'Amico risk category [80]. There have also been reports that bilateral vs. unilateral nerve-sparing in the setting of pT2 disease is associated with a higher rate of PSM, as demonstrated in a series of n = 9915 patients who underwent robotic prostatectomy at two institutions, with relative risk 1.52 [81]. Other studies have not corroborated an increased positive margin rate for intrafascial vs. interfascial nerve-sparing techniques (rate of 9% vs. 9.5%) [82]. The grades of nerve-sparing proposed by Dr. Tewari have been associated with excellent PSM rates, likely owing to preoperative risk stratification based on Gleason score, PSA, digital rectal examination (DRE) findings, cancer volume, and mpMRI findings. The rates of PSM for patients with nerve-sparing grades 1, 2, 3, and 4 were 9.9, 8.1, 7.2, and 8.7%, respectively ($p = 0.636$). The Schatloff series also reported their PSM rate, which was 9% overall. Although the rate of PSM for grade 1 NS was 0%, there was otherwise no consistent correlation between grade of NS and PSM rate (0, 5.7, 16.7, 7.5, 3.6% for grades 1, 2, 3, 4, and 5, respectively), perhaps reflecting good presurgical planning based on patient risk factors [78]. The Veil of Aphrodite technique by the Vattikuti Urology Institute reported a positive margin rate of 13%, which declined to 1.5% for pT2 disease after modification of approach to include en face oversewing of the DVC after apical transection [79].

Regarding the potency rates, it is necessary to standardize the definition of potency, which usually incorporates routine use of oral PDE 5 inhibitors. Furthermore, there is a distinction between restoration of penetrative sexual intercourse vs. return to baseline functioning. There are several contemporary series reporting erectile function outcomes after robotic prostatectomy. Tewari's risk-stratified approach to neural-hammock sparing in n = 2317 men resulted successful intercourse (score of ≥4 on question two of the SHIM and total SHIM >21) of 90.9, 81.4, 73.5, and 62% for nerve-sparing grades 1, 2, 3, and 4, respectively [76]. Regarding return to baseline function: grade 1, 81.7%; grade 2, 74.3%; grade 3, 66.1%; grade 4, 54.5%. Of note, this group also reported earlier return of continence associated with the higher grades of nerve-sparing, which has been controversial [83]. Incidentally, a recent systematic review and meta-analysis of 27 longitudinal cohort studies totaling n = 13,749 patients, however, reported that early urinary continence (at 6 months post-RP) was improved for patients undergoing nerve-sparing vs. non-nerve-sparing surgery (88.9% vs. 69.8%) [84].

Tewari's technical modification of adding real-time penile oxygen monitoring demonstrated that at 6 weeks postoperatively, a larger proportion of patients in the O_2 monitoring group had no ED (24.5% vs. 10.4%, $p < 0.05$) and at 52 weeks this difference was persistent (84% vs. 68%, $p < 0.05$). Furthermore, using the Sexual Health Inventory for Men (SHIM) validated questionnaire at 1 year, a greater number proportion of patients reported minimal to no ED (94% vs. 78%, $p < 0.05$). In this report, the authors did not sub-stratify by grade of nerve sparing [85] (see Section 5.4).

The Schatloff series on grade stratification based on periprostatic arterial anatomy did not report functional outcomes [78]. The Vattikuti Institute series included n = 1142 patients with minimum follow-up of 12 months and among men with normal preoperative function (i.e. SHIM >21) potency rates were 68% in the standard bilateral nerve-sparing patients and 93% in the bilateral Veil nerve-sparing patients [79]. Return to baseline rates depended on preoperative function, and for those without preoperative dysfunction, return to baseline was 39% for standard nerve-sparing and 73% for the Veil technique. Despite these very favorable results, the authors disclosed that only 50% of these patients attained normal SHIM score without medication. Although these findings suggest that the Veil offers improvements in recovery of erectile function, there may be a bias of surgeon experience, as the Veil technique was employed later in the learning curve of this single-surgeon series. This series also demonstrated 84% total urinary control, and 95% social continence (one pad or liner per day) at 12 months follow-up. The role of nerve-sparing in earlier recovery of continence has been corroborated by many series [86–88].

Some limitations of these studies are that they are single institution and often single-surgeon series and there is no direct comparison among different techniques to be able to assess superiority. Furthermore, there may be shortcomings with translation of these techniques into the larger urologic community compared to the immensely high-volume centers where these techniques were invented.

5.4. Intraoperative penile oxygen monitoring

The real-time impact of neurovascular bundle tension on cavernosal ischemia was investigated by Tewari et al. in n = 64 patients [85]. During robotic prostatectomy, these patients underwent real-time penile oxygen monitoring with the Odissey Tissue Oximeter probe placed 2 cm from the base of the penis. Surgical dissection was altered whenever the O_2 alarm sounded until oxygenation was restored to 85%. Functional outcomes were compared to a propensity-matched historical control group of n = 192 patients (matched for age, preoperative prostate specific antigen (PSA), baseline erectile function, comorbidity status, and extent of nerve-sparing). Steps in the operation associated with significant decline in tissue oxygenation included opening the endopelvic fascia, all of the nerve-sparing, excessive traction on the Foley catheter, seminal vesicles, or prostate during the apical dissection, and control of the dorsal vein complex (DVC) prior to apical dissection. Of note, control of the DVC if done after apical transection was not associated with significant penile ischemia. At 6 weeks postoperatively, a larger proportion of patients in the O_2 monitoring group had no ED (24.5% vs. 10.4%, $p < 0.05$) and at 52 weeks this difference was persistent (84% vs. 68%, $p < 0.05$). Furthermore, using the Sexual Health Inventory for Men (SHIM) validated questionnaire at 1 year, a greater number proportion of patients reported minimal to no ED (94% vs. 78%, $p < 0.05$). These findings provide clinical evidence for the importance of minimizing neurovascular bundle manipulation during robotic prostatectomy as a means of preventing neurapraxia/axonotmesis.

Similar evidence comes from a well-designed prospective, randomized, single-blinded study of n = 61 with normal preoperative erectile function from 6 centers [89]. Patients underwent robotic prostatectomy with traditional bilateral nerve sparing compared to nerve-sparing using the Cavermap Surgical Aid. A 12 months post-op, the Cavermap group had mean 15.9 minutes of greater than 60% nocturnal tumescence vs. 2.1 minutes as measured by the

RigiScan. The sexual function inventory questionnaire (SFIQ) scores at 12 months were not significantly different, however. Among those patients with intact response to nerve stimulation after nerve-sparing, 68% of those with bilateral response had recovery on SFIQ vs. 27% with unilateral response, and 0% with no response [89]. A subsequent multi-institutional study utilizing the Cavermap by five experienced surgeons demonstrated limited specificity to identify the precise location of the cavernous nerves, thus limiting its routine application during radical prostatectomy [90].

5.5. No countertraction technique

The detrimental impact of nerve traction injury may also be limited. A series emphasizing nerve-sparing with a lack of countertraction has been published (**Figure 10**). Kowalcyzk et al. reported statistical significantly different erectile function at 5 months post-robotic prostatectomy (24.9% vs. 18.4%, $p = 0.004$), which was confirmed in the multivariable regression model. These differences were no longer present at 12 months (34.7% vs. 33.5%, $p = 0.849$), independent of preoperative erectile function, laterality of nerve sparing, and inter- vs. intrafascial approach [91]. Therefore, "tractionless" surgery may accelerate functional return.

5.6. Minimizing use of electrocautery/thermal energy

In the early experience of robotic prostatectomy, many centers performed dissection of the neurovascular bundle with electrocautery. Ahlering et al. demonstrated slower return of erection function as measured by the IIEF-5 and two questions on the EPIC questionnaire. Of the $n = 125$ patients, only 36 met their inclusion criteria, (age < 66 and IIEF-5 score 22–25), with $n = 3$ having had monopolar electrocautery and $n = 33$ having had bipolar cautery. Of note men with Gleason 7–10 and high volume disease had ipsilateral wide excision of the NVB. Although there was no comparison group, erectile function recovery was modest especially when compared to modern historical series. Among those who had bilateral nerve-sparing, recovery at 15 months was 44.4% and at 24 months was 67.9% [31]. These findings help to support the clinical principle of avoidance of thermal energy during dissection of the neurovascular bundle.

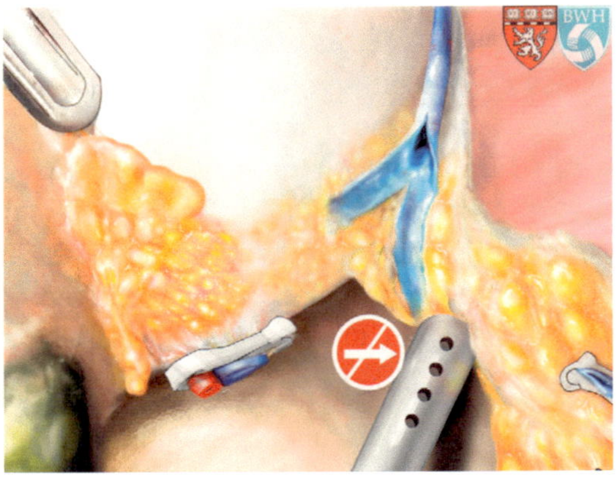

Figure 10. Technique of nerve-sparing with assistant suction neurovascular bundle countertraction which is avoided in the Kowalcyzk et al. technique of nerve-sparing. Reprinted from Kowalczyk et al. [91].

5.7. Seminal vesicle preservation

Building on several observational studies [92, 93], Gilbert et al. reported a randomized controlled, Phase II trial of n = 140 men who underwent radical prostatectomy [94]. Seminal vesicle-sparing approach was employed in 71 men. At 6 and 12 months post-operatively, sexual and urinary function scores were similar on the EPIC questionnaire (erections firm enough for intercourse in 67.7% vs. 56.3%, p = 1). In addition, positive surgical margin status and 12-month biochemical recurrence rates were similar. This approach has understandably not been widely adopted.

5.8. Hypothermic robotic radical prostatectomy

Finley et al. reported the potential benefit of regional hypothermia/cold dissection of the neurovascular bundle in a case–control study of n = 115 who underwent robotic prostatectomy [95, 96]. The rationale for the endeavor mirrors developments in neurosurgery and cardiac surgery that have established significant benefits in randomized studies. Hypothermia was employed to minimize iatrogenic tissue inflammation and consequent cellular edema, lactic acidosis, nerve conduction blockade, free radical damage, and apoptosis that characterizes damage to muscle and nervous tissue. Cold intracorporeal irrigation was employed along with an endorectal cooling balloon cycled with saline at 4°C. Potency rates at 12-months were favorable. Patients subjected to hypothermia were compared to a historical cohort of n = 667 patients. Temperature probes monitored the endorectal and intracorporeal temperatures, which declined to mean 18.7 and 25.6°C, respectively. Potency was assessed during validated questionnaires and defined as "erections adequate for penetration" and "were the erections satisfactory." Potency at 3 months was similar, but at 15 months, the hypothermic group had significantly better function (83% vs. 66%, p = 0.045). There were no differences in oncologic outcomes and no complications related to the technology [97]. These results need further multi-institutional investigation.

5.9. Clipless antegrade nerve preservation

Rather than perform the nerve-sparing in the conventional antegrade (base to apex) fashion, some centers have described a medial to lateral approach. After division of the posterior bladder neck, the posterior plane along the prostate is developed toward the prostatic apex in the midline. The dissection proceeded laterally to release the vascular pedicles and neurovascular bundles in a medial to lateral direction, with sparing use of bipolar cautery. No monopolar cautery or clips were used. Chien et al. reported their series of n = 56 patients who underwent robotic prostatectomy using this approach between 2003 and 2004 [97]. Their outcome metrics relied on the Rand Medical Outcomes Study 36-Item Health Survey, version 2, as well as the University of California, Los Angeles, Prostate Cancer Index up to 12 months postop. Return to baseline potency (allowed use of oral phosphodiesterase inhibitors) among patients with bilateral nerve-sparing occurred in 69%. The positive surgical margin rate in this series was similar to other published techniques at 10.7% [97].

5.10. Intraoperative frozen section analysis

There have been multiple reports of the utility of intraoperative frozen section to allow for more aggressive nerve-sparing in patients whose risk factors may have otherwise prompted a non-nerve sparing surgical approach. In an open series of n = 608 patients who underwent RP, 83 patients were found to have a palpable lesion close to the prostatic capsule [98]. A 4 cm wedge of tissue was excised in the suspicious area for intraoperative frozen section (IOFS). A total of 93% of these IOFS were positive for carcinoma, and 36% of these were pT3. Final positive margin rate overall was 16%. This real-time decision-making allowed for ipsilateral nerve-sparing in 52% of the cases without a negative impact on PSM. Of note, there was a false positive PSM rate of 17%. The applicability to the modern era of robotic prostatectomy may not be lost, but would be based on gross visual suspicion of tumor violation during nerve-sparing.

Another center has pioneered the Neurovascular Structure-Adjacent Frozen-section Examination ("NeuroSAFE") approach to nerve sparing [99]. In this technique, a bilateral nerve-sparing procedure is performed and then the prostate gland is promptly extracted from the surgical field and whole gland circumferential frozen section analysis is performed. The original series consisted of n = 11,069 who underwent open RRP from 2002 to 2011, n = 5392 of whom had the NeuroSAFE technique. When a margin was found to be positive, the ipsilateral neurovascular bundle was resected, including the rectolateral component of the Denonvilliers' fascia, prior to the vesicourethral anastomosis. The sensitivity and specificity of this approach was 93.5 and 98.8%, respectively, with accuracy of 97.3%. Of the 25% found to have PSM initially, 85% of these were converted to final negative margin. False negatives occurred in 2.5% and all of these margins were < 0.5 mm. There were significant reductions in PSM rates within each pathologic tumor stage (except for pT3b) and an increase in the rate of nerve-sparing for all stages. Of note processing time took about 35 minutes and there was no delay in surgery, as hemostasis, bladder closure, lymph node dissection, and posterior reconstruction could be performed during this time (**Figure 11**) [99].

This technique has been translated into robotic surgery in n = 1570 patients from 2004 to 2012, in whom n = 1178 had the NeuroSAFE technique. Intraoperative blood loss was equivalent and nerve-sparing rate increased significantly (overall 97% vs. 81%; pT2 99% vs. 90%; pT3a 94% vs. 74%; pT3b 91% vs. 30%). Furthermore, rate of PSM improved with NeuroSAFE (overall 16% vs. 24%; pT2 8% vs. 15%; pT3a 22% vs. 39%; pT3b 49% vs. 67%; $p < 0.05$) [100]. These findings have contributed to the development of the "Safe-R score," a composite measure of margin status and laterality of nerve sparing [101].

5.11. The influence of surgical modality on nerve-sparing success

It has been postulated that the loss of haptic feedback renders traction-free nerve-sparing difficult during robotic prostatectomy. Conversely, the optical magnification and seven-degrees of freedom afforded by robotic surgery may allow for superior delineation of the neuroanatomy, precision of dissection, and even performance of partial or incremental nerve sparing for patients with concern for locally advanced disease. Such patients may have otherwise been subjected to a non-nerve-sparing technique. Tewari et al. reported earlier return of 50% erectile function (as reported on the EPIC questionnaire) after robotic prostatectomy vs. RRP (mean 180 days vs. 440 days, $p < 0.05$) and earlier return to intercourse (340 days vs. >700 days, $p < 0.05$) Interestingly, these findings were shown even in the setting of a greater number of patients post-RRP using sildenafil (65% vs. 42%) [102]. Such findings were also corroborated by a prospective, non-randomized trial of robotic prostatectomy vs. RRP in n = 208 patients from 2006 to 2007. At

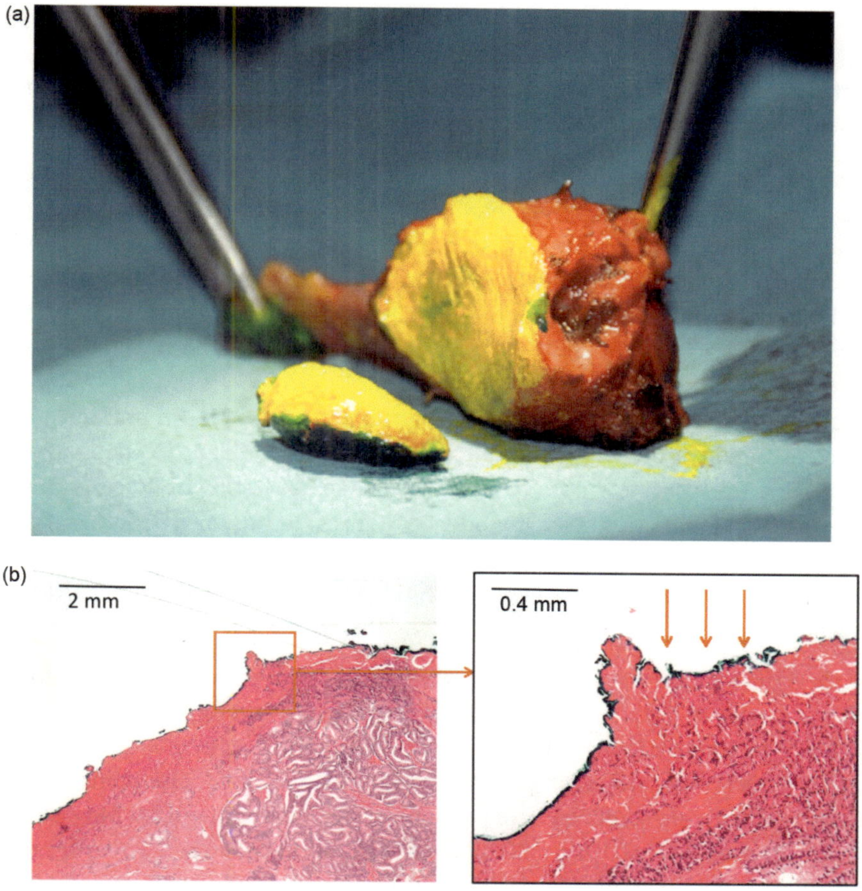

Figure 11. A. Intraoperative picture of NeuroSAFE technique. B. Intraoperative frozen section with tumor contact at linked surface. Reprinted from Beyer et al. [100].

12 months follow-up, of the patients with bilateral nerve-sparing, those who underwent the robotic procedure had superior recovery of erectile function on the IIEF-5 questionnaire (81% vs. 49%, $p < 0.001$) [62]. Further contemporary evidence comes from a systematic review and meta-analysis of 31 studies published between 2008 and 2011 totaling n = 3491 patients [63]. Outcome measures of erectile function were heterogeneous, with some studies employing SHIM > 21 and others using "erections sufficient for intercourse." Cumulative analyses of the six studies with suitable follow-up demonstrated better 12-month potency rates after robotic surgery vs. RRP (24.2% vs. 47.8%; odds ratio 2.84, $p = 0.002$). Absolute risk reduction was 23.6%. Furthermore, 24-month potency was 84% vs. 47% (odds ratio 6.01; $p < 0.001$) Comparison between robotic and laparoscopic approaches was not significant (39.8% vs. 55.6%, $p = 0.21$).

These comparisons may be hampered by different definitions and metrics for erectile dysfunction, patient selection for surgery, and variations in post-operative penile rehabilitation at different institutions. Further evidence is forthcoming from the first randomized controlled phase 3 study of robotic vs. open prostatectomy conducted by Yaxley et al. out of Australia [103]. Although the study randomized n = 326 men and plans to report on urinary and sexual function outcomes (via the EPIC and IIEF questionnaires) at 6 and 12 weeks, as well as 24 months, published results are immature at 12 weeks only. There were no significantly different urinary or sexual function scores at 6 and 12 weeks, nor were there differences in health reported quality of life.

A counterargument to the benefits afford by robotic surgery, however, states that more aggressive nerve sparing, although technically feasible, may not be oncologically safe, given the risk of positive margins. Indeed, the Preston et al. study revealed that positive margins were more likely in patients treated with robotic surgery (relative risk 1.76) compared to open surgery, while there was no difference between lap and robotic surgery [81]. These findings were not corroborated in a very large, albeit retrospective, multi-institutional, multi-national study of n = 22,393 patients, however, which found the lowest rate of positive margins in robotic prostatectomy (13.8%) vs. laparoscopic (16.3%) vs. open (22.8%) [104]. A recent systematic review and meta-analysis by Novara et al. of 21 studies totaling n = 19,238 patients reported similar PSM rates among robotic, laparoscopic, and open surgery, both overall and when sub-stratified into pT2 patients (mean 15%, range 6.5–32% [105]. More recent evidence to mitigate this controversy comes from the previously referenced randomized Phase 3 trial of open vs. robotic prostatectomy by Yaxley et al. Oncologic outcome were equivalent between the two groups, including PSM overall, and for pT2 and pT3 patients (15% vs. 10%, 3% vs. 2%, 11% vs. 8%, respectively) [103].

One notable difference between the open and robotic approach is the use of a retrograde vs. antegrade approach to the dissection of the neurovascular bundle. There is a theoretically reduced risk of placing a clip across the neurovascular bundle with the retrograde approach, which releases the bundle from the prostate prior to obtaining vascular control [106]. These different approaches were compared in a propensity-matched series of n = 344 patients undergoing robotic prostatectomy. Using validated questionnaires at 3,6, and 9 months, the potency rate was significantly higher after the retrograde approach (92.9% vs. 72.1% at 9 months), and this finding was maintained with multivariable analysis. Of note, the PSM rate was similar between groups (11.6% vs. 7%, $p > 0.05$) [107]. Of note, this was a single-surgeon series and the approaches were performed in an interfascial manner, which may not reflect the most current understanding of the cavernous neuroanatomy. Also, the retrograde approach was generally performed more recently in the series with possible artifactual enhancement in outcome from being later in the learning curve. Furthermore, the seemingly excellent results from either approach in this series are likely a consequence of the permissive definition of erection function (erections firm enough for penetration in >50% of attempts).

Of note, although intriguing to consider if there are any technical advantages to nerve sparing with an extraperitoneal vs. transperitoneal approach to robotic prostatectomy, the extant literature has thus far focused exclusively on perioperative rather than functional outcomes [108, 109].

6. Penile rehabilitation

Several options for penile rehabilitation have been proposed and investigated, including pharmacotherapy with oral phosphodiesterase inhibitors or penile intracavernosal injection, as well as use of a vacuum erection device and penile constrictive ring. Often a multimodality approach is advocated. Compliance with these recommendations depends on myriad factors, including physician counseling, patient motivation, and even socioeconomic status—as many of the therapies are not covered under health insurance. The PCOS trial reported that 43% of men tried sildenafil, 25% tried a vacuum erection device, and 17% tried intracavernous injections [52]. Admittedly, the denominator of men who were actually offered these treatments is not known.

The rationale for these treatments has been investigated in preclinical models. There is indeed precedent for treatment success in animal models of chronic low-dose tadalafil administration, with increased cavernosal smooth muscle, decreased fibrous tissue, and functional enhancement of erectile function [110–112]. Similar findings have been reported for sildenafil after bilateral cavernosal nerve damage in a rat model. Nerve damage resulted in elevation in several pro-inflammatory cytokines (interleukin-1β, transforming growth factor β) and markers of oxidative stress (nicotinamide adenine dinucleotide phosphate [NADPH] oxidase, myeloperoxidase, inducible nitric oxide synthase, tumor necrosis factor receptor superfamily member 5 [CD40]), which then normalized after administration of sildenafil in the drinking water. Levels were measured by polymerase chain reaction (PCR) and proteome expression of pelvic ganglia neurons [113].

6.1. Mechanotherapy

The vacuum erection device often in conjunction with penile constrictive ring are routinely recommended for use to assist with recovery of potency after radical prostatectomy. This therapy not only allows for tumescence and penetration, but also cavernosal sinus expansion, smooth muscle "stretching," and mitigation of hypoxia when used on a regular basis [114, 115]. Compared to pharmacotherapies—which are often not covered by the patient's health insurance—VED may be more cost-effective, with a decreased side effect profile and the opportunity for the patient and his partner to take an active role in convalescence. In addition, the mechanism of action does not require intact cavernous nerves for success. There have been multiple retrospective studies examining the impact of the VED [115–117]. These suggest improvement in return of spontaneous erections. In particular, a retrospective study of n = 203 patients who underwent robotic radical prostatectomy between 2007 and 2011 investigated whether PD5I alone, VED alone, or a combination of the two yielded the highest improvement of the SHIM questionnaire, substratified into three groups of baseline EF (SHIM 8–16, SHIM 17–21, SHIM 22–25). For each of the baseline EF groups the combination therapy resulted in the highest proportion of successful potency (erections suitable for penetration) and with the shortest latency period [118].

Randomized evidence comes from Raina et al., who reported on n = 109 patient who underwent open RP (both NS and non-NS) randomized post-op to daily VED therapy vs. observation. Compliance with the device was 80% with 55% partner satisfaction rate. After 9 months of treatment IIEF-5 score was significantly increased for both the NS and non-NS patients compared to the no treatment group. Furthermore, decreased penile length was reported in 63% of the control group vs. 23% among patients who responded to VED treatment [115].

Regarding timing of therapy, earlier initiation of 10 minutes daily VED therapy (1 month post-op vs. at 6 months) has been shown in a small randomized trial of n = 28 men to be superior in terms of 1. IIEF score at 3- and 6-months, and 2. preservation of stretched penile length (vs. 2 cm mean decrease observed in the delayed therapy group) [119].

6.2. Pharmacotherapy

The majority of penile rehabilitation studies incorporate early post-op therapy. Phosphodiesterase type 5 inhibitors have been demonstrated to be effective for the treatment of erectile dysfunction through their inhibitory effect on the enzyme that degrades cGMP. These medications augment the nitric oxide-mediation erectile response through increased relaxation of the cavernosal sinus smooth muscle [120]. The commercially available medications have different half-lives of activity, with Tadalafil being the longest ($T_{1/2}$ sildenafil 3–5 mg; vardenafil 4–5 hours; tadalafil 17.5 hours) [121]. There is also experience with both intraurethral and intracavernosal prostaglandin E, which act via a cAMP-related mechanism to effect cavernosal smooth muscle dilatation [122]. Montorsi et al. published the first randomized, placebo controlled trial in 1997, involving intracavernosal injection of alprostadil three times per week × 12 weeks beginning 1 month after open RP [23]. Newer formulations of intracavernosal therapy include Trimix (prostaglandin, phentolamine—a non-selective alpha-blocker—and papaverine—a non-selective PDE5 inhibitor—and Bimix (papaverine and phentolamine). Given the invasive nature of ICI—as well as the putative higher complication rate regarding pain, hematoma, penile plaque formation, and priapism—this therapy is not universally accepted by patients. Therefore, there is much interest in the oral PDE5 inhibitors as a mechanism of increasing intracavernosal cGMP to promote smooth muscle relaxation and mitigate of the post-RP hypoxic state.

6.2.1. Oral PDE 5 inhibitors

There have been several prospective, randomized studies in this domain, which are summarized **Table 1**. Rationale for these trials was based on findings that daily sildenafil preserves intracorporeal smooth muscle after radical retropubic prostatectomy [123]. The studies tended to exclude men with high grade prostate cancer (i.e. Gleason 8) and those who required adjuvant radiation therapy. Latency of medication initiation is also variable, ranging from time of catheter removal to 4 weeks post op. Based on the cavernous neurotomy rat models in which post-injury cavernous smooth muscle apoptosis begins in 1 day and peaks at 1 week, earlier initiation of treatment has definite clinical rationale [34]. Furthermore, the study end-points are not identical. Some examine the impact on erections during an active treatment phase and others examine the rate of return of spontaneous erections (that is, without the need for pharmacotherapy). The proportion of open vs. robotic RP are also variable (open RP: 39.7–100%). The Jo et al. study out of South Korea is the only study comprised exclusively of patients who underwent robotic prostatectomy, and showed more complete return of erectile function at 12 months with immediate post-catheter removal initiation of 100 mg sildenafil twice weekly compared to waiting until 3 months after surgery [124]. The concomitant use of VED in these studies is not clear, which adds another limitation to their interpretation. Also of interest is a follow-up study to the study by Pavlovich et al. [172] suggesting poorer EPIC scores with nightly sildenafil 50 mg compared to PRN dosing, largely in the urinary irritative and bother subscales of the questionnaire [125]. Further study is required to clarify the implications of this report.

http://dx.doi.org/10.5772/intechopen.79398

Author	Patients	Study drug	Study schema	F/U	Outcome metric	Findings	Conclusion	Limitations
Montorsi et al. [23]	30; mean age 62, "reported satisfactory intercourse preop;" bilateral nerve-sparing	Alprostadil TIW × 12 weeks	Dose titrated for efficacy (2–14 μg) vs. no injection	3 months	"Recovery of spontaneous erections"	80% compliance with injections; 67% recovery vs. 20%	Early ICI with alprostadil increases recovery of spontaneous erections	No sham injection group; no IIEF standardized questionnaire; waited 1 month short f/u; 17% complication
Montorsi et al. [110]	445 (18–64 years); IIEF-EF ≥ 26; bilateral NS; mean age 57.1	Vardenafil × 9 months	10 mg nightly vs. 10 mg PRN within 2 weeks postop	12 months	IIEF-EF ≥ 22 after 2-month washout; then open label PRN	Double blind period: IIEF > 22: 24.8, 32, 48.2% (placebo, nightly, on demand); After 2 months washout and open label PRN no difference	On demand dosing is effective	Did not limit frequency of on demand dosing; dose up to 20 mg
Padma-Nathan et al. [171]	76 (18–70 years) s/p RRP; 8 on Q3 and Q4 of IIEF; mean age 55.5	Sildenafil × 9 months	Nightly 50 mg, 100 mg, placebo within 4 weeks	12 months	IIEF after 8 week washout; plethysmography	IIEF Q3 + Q4 ≥8 and "satisfactory": 4, 26, 29% (placebo, 50 mg, 100 mg)	Sildenafil improved erectile function, but no dose dependence	Closed early for lack of treatment effect; very low rate of EF in placebo arm; waited 4 weeks
Pavlovich et al. [172]	100 (<65 years) s/p MIS RP; IIEF-EF ≥ 26, uni-/bilateral NS; mean age 53.9	Sildenafil × 12 months	50 mg nightly vs. PRN (max 6 per month) immediately after RP	13 months	IIEF, EPIC after 1-mo washout	IIEF-EF > 21: 33.2, 50% (nightly, on demand)	No difference in nightly vs. on demand	No pure placebo arm
Montorsi et al. [173]	423 (≤68 years; IIEF-EF ≥ 22; PSA <10 ng/mL; GS < 8. Bilateral NS; mean age 57.9 years	Tadalafil × 9 months	5 mg daily vs. 20 mg PRN; 6 week washout, then 3 months open-label 5 mg daily	13.5 months	IIEF-EF ≥ 22 after 6-week washout; penile length loss	20.9, 16.9, 19.1% IIEF-EF ≥ 22 (daily, on demand, placebo) after washout—non-signif; 5 mg daily better IIEF-EF vs. placebo	"Unassisted EF was not improved after cessation of active therapy for 9 month." Reduced penile length loss in 5 mg daily (difference 4 mm)	Binary definition of success limited power; patients with mild ED (IIEF-EF 22–25) were included

Author	Patients	Study drug	Study schema	F/U	Outcome metric	Findings	Conclusion	Limitations
Canat et al. [174]	129; mean age 63 years; IIEF-6 no or mild ED; bilateral NS	Tadalafil × 12 weeks	20 mg TIW vs. 20 mg PRN vs. placebo at time of catheter removal	6 weeks, 12 months	IIEF-6 score at 6 weeks and 12 months	6 weeks no diff; 12 months, higher IIEF for TIW group (19.9 vs 15.8 vs. 13.47; TIW, PRN, none)	20 mg TIW is effective and well-tolerated	Lack of placebo
Kim et al. [175]	97; SHIM ≥ 21 and RigiScan >60% × 10 minutes nocturnal erection; b/l NS (robo-, open); mean age 54 years	Sildenafil × 12 months	50 mg starting night after surgery vs. placebo; all patients received 6 tabs × 100 mg/months PRN	13 months	IIEF; RigiScan	RigiScan 40% potency at 13 months for both groups; IIEF > 21 29% vs. 32.4%, non-significant	No difference for 50 mg nightly sildenafil vs. 100 mg PRN	76% compliance; under accrual; lack of true placebo arm
Jo et al. [124]	120; >50 years; IIEF-5 ≥ 17; NS-eligible but not always performed; s/p RALP (~82%);mean age 63.7 years	Sildenafil × 12 months	Sildenafil 100 mg 2×/ week after catheter removal × 3 months; delayed group started at 3 months post-op; then PRN 12 months therapy	12 months	IIEF ≥ 12 months	IIEF ≥ in 41.4% vs. 17.7% (early vs. late); PRN usage similar between groups	Early sildenafil improved full EF recovery during 12 months post-RP	Early group younger (61.7 vs. 65.6); small study

TIW = three times per week; RCT = randomized controlled trial; ICI = intracavernosal injection; f/u = follow-up; NS = nerve sparing; IIEF = International Index of Erectile Function; EF = erectile function; PRN = pro re nata ("on demand"); RRP = radical retropubic prostatectomy; MIS = minimally invasive surgery; RP = radical prostatectomy; EPIC = Expanded prostate cancer index composite; EF = Erectile function; PSA = prostate specific antigen; REF = Residual Erection Function; RALP = robotic-assisted laparoscopic prostatectomy.

Table 1. Randomized controlled trials of post-prostatectomy pharmacologic penile rehabilitation.

A majority of these trials for ED after radical prostatectomy examine daily vs. on-demand dosing schedules. Of note, a randomized, double-blind trial (RESTORE study) in men with mild to moderate ED (IIEF-EF 15–20; *not post-prostatectomy*) of 10 mg vardenafil daily vs. PRN showed no differences in increase of IIEF-EF score [126]. Similar findings appear to be borne out in the post-RP series as well (*see below*). Side effect profiles of the treatment groups were largely favorable and usually without the need for drug discontinuation. Furthermore, daily vs. on demand schedules did not have significantly different adverse effects in a recent meta-analysis, and absolute rates of side effects were not substantially different between treatment and placebo groups overall (59.6% vs. 48.4%) [127]. Side effects generally reported included headache, flushing, dyspepsia, and rhinitis, none of which are severe.

6.2.2. Intraurethral prostaglandin

Intraurethral alprostadil (Medicated Urethral System for Erection, *MUSE*™) has also been developed for use in erectile dysfunction. Experience with this drug for non-post-RP erectile dysfunction has been limited by lack of efficacy and penile pain/dysuria in a large number of patients. Early experience with MUSE after 6 months of post-RP ED showed 55% of the n = 54 patients able to achieve erections suitable for penetration, although only 48% continued long-term therapy (57% of men discontinued therapy for inefficacy) [128]. The author's experience with application of the therapy at 3 weeks post-op for a duration of 6 months showed erections firm enough for penetration in 74% of patients compliant with treatment. All patients reported mild penile pain or urethral burning and 32% of patients discontinued treatment [129].

6.3. Pelvic floor PT

The role of pelvic floor physical therapy (PFMT; "Kegel" exercises) on return of urinary continence has been well understood, as evidenced by meta-analyses demonstrating earlier return of continence with preoperative PMFT and biofeedback [130, 131]. The impact of such therapy on recovery of sexual function has also been explored. Physical therapy efforts focus on the bulbocavernosus (bulbospongiosus) and ischiocavernosus muscles. Contraction of the ischiocavernosus muscle may compress the proximal aspects of the corpora cavernosa and increase intracavernosal pressure during erection [132]. Also, muscle contraction has been shown to increase levels of brain-derived neurotrophic factor in muscle cells, which may have a role in promoting neuronal growth after nerve injury [133]. A trial of n = 55 men with ED for ≥6 months randomized one group to PFMT with biofeedback + lifestyle changes vs. lifestyle changes alone [134]. Lifestyle changes consisted of alcohol intake reduction, smoking cessation, increasing exercise, and avoiding bicycle riding. Outcomes were assessed with IIEF and anal pressure measurements. At 3 months follow-up, the PFMT group had greater improvement in IIEF than the lifestyle changes alone group ($p < 0.001$). Other concomitant therapies for ED (i.e. PDE5 inhibitors or vacuum erection device) were not disclosed by the authors, limiting the strength of the results. Also, there were no post-prostatectomy patients in this cohort.

With regard to prostatectomy, the timing is such physical therapy is also interesting to consider and there is no established consensus of whether pre- and postoperative physical therapy is superior to postoperative therapy alone. Perez et al. examined the use of biofeedback preoperatively to strengthen the levator muscles prior to radical prostatectomy [135]. Their methods employed a device that provided visual feedback based on intra-anal pressures. In this prospective cohort study, a total of n = 20 patients completed 10 sessions pre-RP and n = 32 patients proceeded directly to surgery. Potency outcomes were assessed using the IIEF-5, although follow-up time was not clear. The erectile dysfunction rate in the physical therapy group was 5% vs. 48.6% in the control group < p < 0.001). There are likely variations in physical therapy technique and not all methods are standardized.

The impact of PFMT on erectile function after radical prostatectomy has also been examined. Prota et al. studied n = 52 patients who underwent open RP and randomized them to PFMT + biofeedback weekly × 3 months (beginning at time of catheter removal) vs. verbal instructions only [136]. Nerve-sparing was performed in a similar proportion of patients in each group (64.7% vs. 68.8%). There was earlier recovery (IIEF >20) in the treatment group which persisted at 12 months post-op (47.1% vs. 12.5%). The authors report an absolute risk reduction of 34.6%, with number needed to treat (NNT) of 3. These results are even more encouraging given that oral PDE5 inhibitor therapy was withheld during the study. This study provides level 1b evidence supporting the use of post-operative PFMT for erectile function recovery [136]. Optimal schedule and intensity has yet to be determined.

Additional randomized controlled trials are needed to further assess the utility of PFMT in the restoration of potency.

6.4. Novel therapies

6.4.1. Hyperbaric oxygen

The role of hyperbaric oxygen (HBO) in Urology for treatment of radiation-induced hemorrhagic cystitis is well known. Application of this technology to post-RP erectile dysfunction is controversial. There have been preclinical studies in rats with cavernous nerve injury undergoing HBO that demonstrate higher intracavernosal pressure/mean arterial pressure ratio, increased levels of penile nerve growth factor (NGF) and endothelial nitric oxide synthase (eNOS) compared to the controls. Tissue studies on smooth muscle to collagen ratio, however, did not show a significant difference after HBO [137]. Exposure to 100% oxygen at 2 atm pressure induces stem cell differentiation and neovascularization, as well as vasoconstriction that attenuates tissue edema [138]. These findings underlie the rationale for translational studies. Chiles et al. published the first randomized, double-blind controlled trial of HBO vs. air for men after RP [139]. Although the authors were unable to demonstrate significant difference in IIEF score at 18 months, uncertainty about the proper regimen for therapy (total number and frequency of treatments) and lack of a true "sham" group may have limited their ability to detect a clinically relevant difference in outcome.

6.4.2. Neuroprotective agents

There is a growing body of literature on drug therapy to preempt or mitigate the post-cavernosal nerve injury pro-inflammatory environment. The immunophilin ligand FK506 (tacrolimus)—traditionally thought of as an immunosuppressive agent and widely used in for solid organ transplant—has been implicated in a neuroprotective role when administered as early as 1 day following partial nerve-crush injury in a rat model [140]. Further work has demonstrated improved intracavernous pressure/mean arterial pressure ratio, restoration of inducible nitric oxide synthase (iNOS) staining, reduced apoptosis, preservation of cavernosal architecture, and upregulation of glutathione peroxidase (GPX) with resultant decrease in oxidative-stress-induced tissue damage [141, 142].

Pioglitazone, a thiazolidinedione used for the treatment of diabetes mellitus, may enhance neuronal survival and regeneration and decrease inflammation, and has been shown to be neuroprotective in models of sciatic nerve ischemia and optic nerve crush injury, as well as BCNI [143–145]. Furthermore, a small randomized controlled trial has shown efficacy of this agent for erectile dysfunction refractory to sildenafil [146]. A study by Katz et al. investigated the impact of pioglitazone on pelvic ganglion neurons after bilateral cavernosal nerve injury (BCNI) in Sprague-Dawley rats [147]. Four groups were examined: sham surgery, BCNI, BCNI + post-operative pioglitazone, BCNI + pre- and post-operative therapy. Gene expression profiles of neuronal nitric oxide synthase, neurturin, glial cell line-derived neurotrophic factor family receptor alpha-2 (GFRα2), and β-III tubulin were upregulated in the pre-operative therapy group [147]. Further work is necessary to fully explore the utility of this therapy.

6.4.3. Amnion-chorion membrane

Dehydrated human amnion-chorion membrane allograft (dHACM) is a source of implantable neurotrophic factors and cytokines which promote neural survival and facilitate axonal regeneration. Its application has been examined in a rat model of axonal regeneration after spinal cord injury [148]. Clinically, it has been applied in the treatment of burns, corneal injuries, chronic venous ulcers, and chronic wounds [149]. There has been preliminary work in the placement of this membrane after bilateral nerve-sparing robotic RP to accelerate erectile functional recovery after surgery [150]. A single-surgeon propensity-matched analysis of preoperatively potent (SHIM >19) and continent (American Urological Association Symptom Score < 10) patients (n = 58) demonstrated earlier return of continence (1.2 months vs. 1.8 months, p = 0.033) and potency (1.34 months vs. 3.39 months, p = 0.007) with the wrap. (AmnioFix; *MiMedx Group, Marietta, GA, USA*) Some limitations of this series include the small size, lack of randomization, and short mean follow-up of 4 months, which limits conclusions about oncologic safety vis-à-vis risk of biochemical recurrence (BCR). Furthermore, functional recovery rates appear much higher than other series in the literature, and may be a consequence of the recall bias used to assess level of function. These preliminary results are certainly encouraging.

The dHACM allograft wrap was recently examined in a series of n = 940 patients (preoperative SHIM > 20) who underwent robotic RP with bilateral nerve-sparing [151]. A total of n = 235 had bilateral dHACM placement and these were propensity matched in a 1:3 proportion to non-dHACM patients (n = 705). Potency recovery rates were higher in the dHACM group at all time points except 12 months. Time to potency was significantly shorter in the dHACM group after bilateral NS (2.2 months vs. 2.8 months, p = 0.029) and partial NS (3 months vs. 3.9 months). After 12 months follow-up, erections sufficient for penetration were similar. Of note, the recovery rates in this study were higher than what is generally reported in the literature. Also, although the rate of biochemical recurrence at 12 months was similar between groups, longer follow-up is certainly needed to demonstrate the oncologic safety of this application of technology.

A recent pre-clinical study of the role of hemostatic tissue sealing sheets has also investigated the impact on erectile function recovery in a series of 21 Sprague-Dawley rats [152]. The TachoSil (CSL Behring, Tokyo, Japan) is a collagen sponge coated on one side with fibrinogen and thrombin and is approved for achieving hemostasis during surgery. Contact between the sheet and blood or serosanguinous fluid results in deposition of a fibrin clot. Compared to sham surgery, the rats who underwent cavernous nerve dissection and had the TachoSil placed demonstrated similar intracavernous pressure/mean arterial pressure ratios at 4 weeks post-op. Furthermore, PCR-measured expression of inflammatory and oxidative markers (internleukin-6, tumor growth factor beta1, and heme-oxygenase-1) in the major pelvic ganglion was significantly reduced in the sheet group ($p < 0.05$).

6.4.4. *Stem cell therapy*

Stem cells may be harvested from growing embryos (embryonic stem cells) or as allografts from bone marrow or adipose tissue (mesenchymal stem cells). This technology has been applied to rat models of bilateral cavernosal nerve crush injury and shown considerable promise. Bochinski et al. [153] conducted a study of embryonic stem cells induced along the neuronal cell line with brain-derived neurotrophic factor [153]. These stem cells were then injected into the major pelvic ganglion (MPG) (group 3) and into the corpora cavernosa (group 4) of rats after BCNI. The study was well controlled with sham surgery (group 1) as well as a BCNI group with injection of culture media only (group 2). Volume of stem cells injected was 500 μL of a 10,000 cells/mL solution. Erectile response was assessed by electrostimulation of the cavernosal nerve at 3 months. Immunohistochemistry was also performed of the penile tissue to assess levels of nitric-oxide synthase-containing fibers and neurofilament concentration. Intracavernosal pressure in response to electrostimulation was greatest for sham surgery and lowest for group 2, which was also significantly lower than groups 3 and 4. The neurofilament stain of tissue taken from the MPG and the corpus cavernosum was also greater in groups 3 and 4 compared to group 2 (**Figure 12**). Such neurofilaments are involved in establishing tensile strength and putatively intracellular transport guidance to axons and dendrites [154]. The authors conclude that preservation of the neuronal architecture may promote/facilitate nerve regeneration after nerve injury.

There have been several more studies investigating the role of stem cells in BCNI in rats, either alone [155] or in combination with PDE5 inhibitors [156, 157]. Furthermore, Lin et al. reported that adipose-derived stem cells (ADSCs) injected into the corpora cavernosa migrated within days to the bone marrow and then to the MPG [158]. Subsequent work has been reexamined in multiple systematic reviews and meta-analyses, reiterating the efficacy of these methods in 12 studies, $n = 319$ rats and 20 studies, $n = 248$ rats, respectively [159, 160]. The combination of stem cells + PDE5 inhibitor therapy appears to have the greatest effect [159]. Consistent outcomes among the studies were increase in the ICP/MAP ratio, levels of neuronal nitric oxide synthase, cavernous smooth muscle content, ratio of cavernous smooth muscle to collage, and cGMP levels [160]. Furthermore, stem cells modified by growth or neurotrophic factors

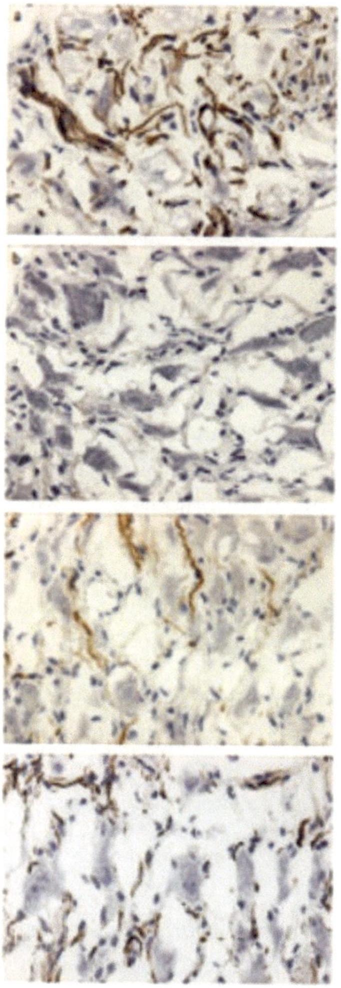

Figure 12. Neurofilament staining in major pelvic ganglion (MPG) of rats after bilateral cavernosal nerve crush injury (BNCI). A. Sham surgery. B. BCNI alone C. BCNI + neuronal stem cells injected into corpora cavernosa. Reprinted from Bochinski et al. [153].

prior to implantation appeared to exert the greatest benefit [160]. Although there are many processing steps to refine and standardize, this approach remains a riveting endeavor in the arena of penile rehabilitation.

7. Penile prosthesis implantation

Despite these advances in the restoration of endogenous erectile function after radical prostatectomy, some men will have dysfunction refractory to the above treatments. The final line treatment option for such patients is insertion of a penile prosthesis, which may in fact be conceived as a type of mechanotherapy. This procedure eliminates the possibility of any spontaneous erectile function in the future and has many potential complications, including pain, erosion, extrusion, infection, mechanical failure, need for revision, and altered penile sensation. There have been a number of surgical improvements that have reduced the infection rate, including the "no touch" technique, standardized protocols for perioperative antibiotics, and the development of antibiotic-impregnated and hydrophilic devices [161–164]. Although the technique of 3-piece penile prosthesis insertion is beyond the scope of this chapter, there are a number of considerations with regard to radical prostatectomy. The cavernosal smooth muscle fibrosis and penile shortening can have an impact on the size of the cylinders able to be accommodated by the corpora, leading to actual or perceived reduction in penile length. Furthermore, the lack of glans tumescence with cylinder expansion may exacerbate the perceived loss of size. After appropriate dilation of the corporal bodies with the dilators, fibrosis should not preclude placement of a three-piece inflatable prosthesis, which has been reported to have the highest satisfaction rates and lowest rate of mechanical failure [165]. Some models of the 3-piece prosthesis (i.e. American Medical Systems, AMS 700 CX) allow for cylinder axial expansion to allow girth. This is important for men with penile plaques/Peyronie's disease and penile curvature that must be corrected during placement of the prosthesis [164]. Although not previously discussed, Peyronie's disease is another "sexual" complication of radical prostatectomy, thought to be from repetitive "buckling" injury to the phallus as a result of intercourse in the setting of an incomplete erection.

Reservoir placement during the three-piece prosthesis surgery also deserves consideration, given the previous dissection of the space of Retzius during the prostatectomy. Given the increased risk of bladder perforation, bowel and vascular injury in this setting, some authors favor ectopic reservoir placement just posterior to the rectus muscle and anterior to the transversalis fascia [166, 167]. Single-institution series have reported excellent outcomes with this approach [166, 167].

Satisfaction with this treatment appears favorable, as exemplified in a recent study of n = 71 patients who underwent penile prosthesis implantation after radical prostatectomy [168]. Pillay et al. employed the EDITS and SEAR questionnaires, as well as the Prostate Cancer-Related Quality of Life Scale and Patient Health Questionnaire-9 (PHQ-9) for both patients and their partners. They reported good sexual function (EPID score > 60) in 77% of men and treatment satisfaction in 94% (EDITS score > 50). Other studies have actually reported improved satisfaction for men undergoing early penile prosthesis insertion compared to those receiving sildenafil or intracavernosal injection therapy 6 months after radical prostatectomy [169, 170]. Such studies did not employ early aggressive pharmacologic penile rehabilitation programs, however. Certainly, for the appropriately selected patient, penile prosthesis implantation has a very high level of success and satisfaction for patients and their partners alike.

8. Conclusions

There have been many advances in the understanding of erectile dysfunction as a result of radical prostatectomy since the initial pioneering work by Walsh & Donker almost 40 years ago. Refined understanding of neuroanatomy, beneficial modifications in surgical technique, the advent of robotic surgery, and the exploration of pre- and post-operative rehabilitation techniques using mechanotherapy and pharmaceuticals have improved the prognosis for potency recovery after this once morbid surgery. Further developments in the realm of local and systemic therapies for cavernous nerve neuroprotection and regeneration may mitigate the cascade of cavernosal smooth muscle apoptosis, fibrosis, and veno-occlusive dysfunction that jeopardizes further erectile function recovery after the period of post-operative neurapraxia. Achievement of the Trifecta is extremely important to patients and clinicians alike, and will surely inspire the future waves of investigations that continue to elucidate this field.

Conflict of interest

I have no conflicts of interest to disclose.

Notes/Thanks/Other declarations

None.

Author details

Michael Whalen

Address all correspondence to: mwhalen@mfa.gwu.edu

Department of Urology, George Washington University School of Medicine and Health Sciences, Washington, DC, USA

References

[1] Nandipati K, Raina R, Agarwal A, et al. Erectile dysfunction following radical retropubic prostatectomy: Epidemiology, pathophysiology and pharmacological management. Drugs & Aging. 2006;**23**(2):101-117

[2] Molodysky E, Liu SP, Huang SJ, Hus GJ. Penile vascular surgery for treating erectile dysfunction: Current role and future direction. Arab Journal of Urology. 2013;**11**(3):254-266. Available from: https://creativecommons.org/licenses/by-nc-nd/3.0/

[3] Rogers CG, Trock BP, Walsh PC. Preservation of accessory pudendal arteries during radical retropubic prostatectomy: Surgical technique and results. Urology. Jul 2004; **64**(1):148-151

[4] Mulhall JP, Secin FP, Guillonneau B. Artery sparing radical prostatectomy—Myth or reality? The Journal of Urology. 2008;**179**(3):827-831

[5] Saenz de Tejada I, Goldstein I, Azadzoi K, et al. Impaired neurogenic and endothelium-mediated relaxation of penile smooth muscle from diabetic men with impotence. The New England Journal of Medicine. 1989;**320**:1025-1030

[6] Walsh PC, Donker PJ. Impotence following radical prostatectomy: Insight into etiology and prevention. The Journal of Urology. 1982;**128**:492-497

[7] Walsh PC, Lepor H, Eggleston JC. Radical prostatectomy with preservation of sexual function: Anatomical and pathological considerations. Prostate. 1983;**4**:473-485

[8] Costello AJ, Brooks M, Cole OJ. Anatomical studies of the neurovascular bundle and cavernosal nerves. BJU International. 2004;**94**(7):1071-1076

[9] Walz J, Burnett AL, Costello AJ, Eastham JA, Graefen M, Guillonneau B, et al. A critical analysis of the current knowledge of surgical anatomy related to optimization of cancer control and preservation of continence and erection in candidates for radical prostatectomy. European Urology. 2010;**57**:179-192

[10] Lunacek A, Schwentner C, Fritsch H, et al. Anatomical radical retropubic prostatectomy 'curtain dissection' of the neurovascular bundle. BJU International. 2005;**95**:1226-1231

[11] Menon M, Shrivastava A, Bhandari M, et al. Vattikuti institute prostatectomy: Technical modifications in 2009. European Urology. 2009;**56**:89-96

[12] Tewari A, Takenaka A, Mtui E, et al. The proximal neurovascular plate and the tri-zonal neural architecture around the prostate gland: Importance in the athermal robotic technique of nerve-sparing prostatectomy. BJU International. 2006;**98**(2):314-323

[13] Eichelberg C, Erbersdobler A, Michl U, et al. Nerve distribution along the prostatic capsule. European Urology. 2007;**51**:105-110

[14] Lee SB, Hong SK, Choe G, et al. Periprostatic distribution of nerves in specimens from non-nerve-sparing radical retropubic prostatectomy. Urology. 2008;**72**(4):878-881

[15] Takenaka A, Murakami G, Soga H, et al. Anatomical analysis of the neurovascular bundle supplying penile cavernous tissue to ensure a reliable nerve graft after radical prostatectomy. The Journal of Urology. 2004;**172**:1032-1035

[16] Ganzer R, Blana A, Gaumann A, et al. Topographical anatomy of periprostatic and capsular nerves: Quantification and computerized planimetry. European Urology. 2008;**54**(2):353-360

[17] Kaiho Y, Nakagawa H, Saito H, et al. Nerves at the ventral prostatic capsule contribute to erectile function: Initial electrophysiological assessment in humans. European Urology. 2009;**55**:148-154

[18] Costello AJ, Dowdle BW, Namdarian B, et al. Immunohistochemical study of the cavernous nerves in the periprostatic region. BJU International. 2011;**107**:1210-1215

[19] Ganzer R, Stolzenburg JU, Wieland WF, et al. Anatomic study of periprostatic nerve distribution: Immunohistochemical differentiation of parasympathetic and sympathetic nerve fibres. European Urology. 2012;**62**:1150-1156

[20] Chen SC, Hsieh CH, Hsu GL, et al. The progression of the penile vein: Could it be recurrent? Journal of Andrology. 2005;**26**:56-63

[21] Mulhall JP, Slovick R, Hotaling J, et al. Erectile dysfunction after radical prostatectomy: Hemodynamic profiles and their correlation with the recovery of erectile function. The Journal of Urology. 2002;**167**:1371-1375

[22] Zelefsky MJ, Eid JF. Elucidating the etiology of erectile dysfunction after definitive therapy for prostate cancer. International Journal of Radiation Oncology, Biology, Physics. 1998;**40**:129-133

[23] Montorsi F, Guazzoni G, Strambi LF, et al. Recovery of spontaneous erectile function after nerve-sparing radical retropubic prostatectomy with and without early intracavernous injections of alprostadil: Results of a prospective randomized trial. The Journal of Urology. 1997;**158**:1408-1410

[24] Stanford JL, Fend Z, Hamilton AS, et al. Urinary and sexual function after radical prostatectomy for clinically localized prostate cancer: The prostate cancer outcomes study. Journal of the American Medical Association. 2000;**283**:354-360

[25] Kilminster S, Muller S, Menon M, et al. Predicting erectile function outcome in men after radical prostatectomy for prostate cancer. BJU International;**110**:422-426

[26] Parvizi J, Kim GK. Nerve injuries related to orthopaedics. High Yield Orthopaedics. 2010;**154**:317-219

[27] Nakata DA, Stoelting RK. Postoperative peripheral neuropathy. In: Complications in Anesthesia. 2nd ed. Vol. 221. 2007. pp. 881-884

[28] Gonzalez-Perez F, Udina E, Navarro X. Extracellular matrix components in peripheral nerve regeneration. International Review of Neurobiology. 2013;**108**:257-275

[29] Navarro X, Vivo M, Valero-Cabre A. Neural plasticity after peripheral nerve injury and regeneration. Progress in Neurobiology. 2007;**82**(4):163-201

[30] Ong AM, Su LM, Varkarakis I, et al. Nerve sparing radical prostatectomy: Effects of hemostatic energy sources on the recovery of cavernous nerve function in a canine model. The Journal of Urology. 2004;**172**(4 Pt 1):1318-1322

[31] Ahlering TE, Eichel L, Skarecky D. Evaluation of long-term thermal injury using cautery during nerve sparing robotic prostatectomy. Urology. 2008;**72**:1371-1374

[32] Klein LT, Miller MI, Buttyan R, et al. Apoptosis in the rat penis after penile denervation. The Journal of Urology. 1997;**158**:626-630

[33] Moreland RB. Is there a role of hypoxemia in penile fibrosis: A viewpoint presented to the Society for the Study of impotence. International Journal of Impotence Research. 1998;**10**:113-120

[34] User HM, Hairston JH, Zelner DJ, et al. Penile weight and cell subtype specific changes in a post-radical prostatectomy model of erectile dysfunction. The Journal of Urology. 2003;**169**:1175-1179

[35] Hatzimouratidis K, Burnett AL, Hatzichristou D, et al. Phosphodiesterase type 5 inhibitors in postprostatectomy erectile dysfunction: A critical analysis of the basic science rationale and clinical application. European Urology. 2009;**55**(2):334-347

[36] de Groat, WC and Booth, AM. Neural control of penile erection. In: The Autonomic Nervous System, Vol. 3, Nervous Control of the Urogenital System, ed. CA Maggi. Chur, Switzerland: Harwood Academic Publishers, pp. 467-524

[37] Cellek S. Nitrergic-noradrenergic interaction in penile erection: A new insight into erection dysfunction. Drugs Today. 2000;**36**(2-3):135-146

[38] Saenz de Tejada I, Kim NN, Goldstein I, et al. Regulation of pre-synaptic alpha adrenergic activity in the corpus cavernosum. International Journal of Impotence Research. 2000;**12**(Suppl 1):S20-S25

[39] Dausse JP, Leriche A, Yoblonsky F. Patterns of messenger mRNA expression for alpha-1 adrenoceptor subtypes in human corpus cavernosum. The Journal of Urology. 1998;**160**:597-600

[40] Martinez-Salamanca JI, La Fuente JM, Fernandez A, et al. Nitrergic function is lost but endothelial function is preserved in the corpus cavernosum and penile resistance arteries of men after radical prostatectomy. The Journal of Sexual Medicine. 2015;**12**:590-599

[41] Martinez-Salamanca JI, La Fuente JM, Martinez-Salamanca E, et al. α1A-adrenergic receptor antagonism improves erectile and cavernosal responses in rats with cavernous nerve injury and enhances neurogenic responses in human corpus cavernosum from patients with erectile dysfunction secondary to radical prostatectomy. The Journal of Sexual Medicine. 2016;**13**(12):1844-1857

[42] Johannes CB, Araujo AB, Feldman HA, et al. Incidence of erectile dysfunction in men 40-69 years old: Longitudinal results from the Massachusetts Male Aging Study. The Journal of Urology. 2000;**163**:460-463

[43] Laumann EO, Gagnon JH, Michael RT, Michaels S. National Health and Social Life Survey. Ann Arbor, MI, United States: Inter-university Consortium for Political and Social Research [distributor]; 1992 [Apr 17, 2008]. DOI: 10.3886/ICPSR06647.v2

[44] Lewis RW, Rugl-Meyer KS, Bosch R, et al. Epidemiology/risk factors of sexual dysfunction. The Journal of Sexual Medicine. 2004;**1**(1):35-39

[45] Rosen RC, Riley A, Wagner G, et al. The international index of erectile function (IIEF): A multidimensional scale for assessment of erectile dysfunction. Urology. 1997; **49**(6):822-830

[46] Rosen RC, Cappelleri JC, Gendrano N. The international index of erectile function (IIEF): A state-of-the-science review. International Journal of Impotence Research. 2002; **14**:226-244

[47] Rosen RC, Cappelleri JC, Smith MD, et al. Development and evaluation of an abridged, 5-item version of the international index of erectile function (IIEF-5) as a diagnostic tool for erectile dysfunction. International Journal of Impotence Research. 1999;**11**(6):319-326

[48] Cappelleri JC, Siegel RL, Glasser DB, et al. Relationship between patient self-assessment of erectile dysfunction and the sexual health inventory for men. Clinical Therapeutics. 2001;**23**(10):1707-1719

[49] Althof SE, Corty EW, Levine SB, et al. EDITS: Development of questionnaires for evaluation satisfaction with treatments for erectile dysfunction. Urology. 1999;**53**(4):793-799

[50] Cappelleri JC, Stecher VJ. An assessment of patient-reported outcomes for men with erectile dysfunction: Pfizer's perspective. International Journal of Impotence Research. 2008;**20**(4):343-357

[51] Wei JT, Dunn RL, Litwinn MS, et al. Development and validation of the expanded prostate cancer index composite (EPIC) for comprehensive assessment of health-related quality of life in men with prostate cancer. Urology. 2000;**56**(6):899-905

[52] Penson DF, McLerran D, Feng Z, et al. 5-year urinary and sexual outcome after radical prostatectomy: Results from the prostate cancer outcome study. The Journal of Urology. 2005;**173**:1701-1705

[53] Resnick MJ, Koyama T, Fan KH, et al. Long-term functional outcomes after treatment for localized prostate cancer. New England Journal of Medicine. 2013;**368**:436-445

[54] Salonia Z, Zanni G, Gallina A, et al. Baseline potency in candidates for bilateral nerve-sparing radical retropubic prostatectomy. European Urology. 2006;**50**:360-365

[55] Dubbelman YD, Dohle GR, Schroder FH. Sexual function before and after radical retropubic prostatectomy: A systematic review of prognostic indicators for a successful outcome. European Urology. 2006;**50**(4):711-718

[56] Kundu SD, Roehl KA, Eggener SE, et al. Potency, continence and complications in 3477 consecutive radical retropubic prostatectomies. The Journal of Urology. 2004; **172**:2227-2231

[57] Geary ES, Dendinger TE, Freiha FS, et al. Nerve sparing radical prostatectomy: A different view. The Journal of Urology. 1995;**154**:145-149

[58] Walsh PC, Marschke P, Ricker D, et al. Patient-reported urinary continence and sexual function after anatomic radical prostatectomy. Urology. 2002;**55**:58-61

[59] Tsujimura A, Matsumiya K, Miyagawa Y, et al. Relation between erectile dysfunction and urinary incontinence after nerve-sparing and non-nerve sparing radical prostatectomy. Urologia Internationalis. 2004;**73**:31-35

[60] Rabbani F, Stepleton AMF, Kattan MW, et al. Factors predicting recovery of erections after radical prostatectomy. The Journal of Urology. 2000;**164**:1929-1934

[61] Hu JC, Elkin EP, Pasta DJ, et al. Predicting quality of life after radical prostatectomy: Results from CaPSURE. The Journal of Urology. 2004;**171**:703-707

[62] Ficarra V, Novara G, Fracalanza S, et al. A prospective, non-randomized trial comparing robot-assisted laparoscopic and retropubic radical prostatectomy in one European institution. BJU International. 2009;**104**:534-539

[63] Ficarra V, Novara G, Ahlering TE, et al. Systematic review and meta-analysis of studies reporting potency rates after robot-assisted radical prostatectomy. European Urology. 2012;**62**(3):418-430

[64] Zorn KC, Wille MA, Thong AE, et al. Continued improvement of perioperative, pathological, and continence outcomes during 700 robot-assisted radical prostatectomies. The Canadian Journal of Urology. 2009;**16**:4742-4749

[65] Moskovic DJ, Alphs H, Nelson CJ, et al. Subjective characterization of nerve sparing predicts recovery of erectile function after radical prostatectomy: Defining the utility of a nerve sparing grading system. The Journal of Sexual Medicine. 2011;**8**:255-260

[66] Levinson AW, Pavlovich CP, Ward NT. Association of surgeon subjective characterization of nerve sparing quality with potency following laparoscopic radical prostatectomy. The Journal of Urology. 2008;**179**:1510-1514

[67] McCullough AR. Prevention and management of erectile dysfunction following radical prostatectomy. The Urologic Clinics of North America. 2001;**28**:613-627

[68] Lee JK, Assel M, Thong AE, et al. Unexpected long-term improvements in urinary and erectile function in a large cohort of men with self-reported outcomes following radical prostatectomy. European Urology. 2015;**68**(5):899-905

[69] Abdollah F, Sun M, Suardi N, et al. Prediction of functional outcomes after nerve-sparing radical prostatectomy. Results of conditional survival analysis. European Urology. 2012;**62**:42-42

[70] Glickman L, Godoy G, Lepor H. Changes in continence and erectile function between 2 and 4 years after radical prostatectomy. The Journal of Urology. 2009;**181**:731-735

[71] Siddiqui MM, Rais-Bahrami S, Turkbey B, et al. Comparison of MR/ultrasound fusion-guided biopsy with ultrasound-guided biopsy for the diagnosis of prostate cancer. Journal of the American Medical Association. 2015;**313**(4):390-397

[72] Ahmed HU, Bosaily AES, Brown LC, et al. Diagnostic accuracy of multi-parametric MRI and TRUS biopsy in prostate cancer (Promis): A paired validating confirmatory study. Lancet. 2017;**389**:815-822

[73] Yossepowitch O, Briganti A, Eastham JA, et al. Positive surgical margins after radical prostatectomy: A systematic review and contemporary update. European Urology. 2014;**65**(2):303-313

[74] De Rooij M, Hamoen EHJ, Aitjes JA, et al. Accuracy of magnetic resonance imaging for local staging of prostate cancer: A diagnostic meta-analysis. European Urology. 2016;**70**(2):233-245

[75] Rud E, Baco E, Klotz D, et al. Does preoperative magnetic resonance imaging reduce the rate of positive surgical margins at radical prostatectomy in a randomized clinical trial? European Urology. 2015;**68**(3):487-496

[76] Tewari AK, Srivastava A, Huang MW, et al. Anatomical grades of nerve sparing: A risk-stratified approach to neural-hammock sparing during robot-assisted radical prostatectomy (RARP). BJU International. 2011;**108**:984-992

[77] Ficarra V, Cavalleri S, Novara G, et al. Evidence from robot-assisted laparoscopic radical prostatectomy: A systematic review. European Urology. 2007:45-55

[78] Schatloff O, Chauhan S, Sivaraman A, et al. Anatomic grading of nerve sparing during robot-assisted radical prostatectomy. European Urology. 2012;**61**:796-802

[79] Menon M, Shrivastava A, Kaul S, et al. Vattikuti institute prostatectomy: Contemporary technique and analysis of results. European Urology. 2007;**51**:648-658

[80] Yee DS, Narula N, Amin MB, et al. Robot-assisted radical prostatectomy: Current evaluation of surgical margins in clinically low-, intermediate-, and high-risk prostate cancer. Journal of Endourology. 2009;**23**(9):1461-1465

[81] Preston MA, Breau RH, Lantz AG, et al. The association between nerve-sparing and a positive surgical margin during radical prostatectomy. Urologic Oncology. 2015;**33**(1):18.e1-18.e6

[82] Stolzenburg JU, Kallidonis P, Do M, et al. A comparison of outcomes for interfascial and intrafascial nerve-sparing radical prostatectomy. Urology. 2010;**76**(3):743-748

[83] Srivastava A, Chopra S, Pham A, et al. Effect of a risk-stratified grade of nerve-sparing technique on early return of continence after robot-assisted laparoscopic radical prostatectomy. European Urology. 2013;**63**:438-444

[84] Reeves F, Preece P, Kapoor J, et al. Preservation of the neurovascular bundles is associated with improved time to continence after radical prostatectomy but not long-term continence rates: Results of a systematic review and meta-analysis. European Urology. 2015;**68**(4):692-704

[85] Tewari A, Srivastava A. Sooriakumaran, et al. technique of traction-free nerve sparing robotic prostatectomy: Delicate tissue handling by real-time penile oxygen monitoring. International Journal of Impotence Research. 2012;**24**(1):11-19

[86] Choi WW, Freire MP, Soukup JR, et al. Nerve-sparing technique and urinary control after robot-assisted laparoscopic prostatectomy. World Journal of Urology. 2011;**29**:21-27

[87] Ko YH, Coelho RF, Chauhan S, et al. Factors affecting return of continence 3 months after robot-assisted radical prostatectomy: Analysis from a large, prospective data by a single surgeon. The Journal of Urology. 2012;**187**:190-194

[88] Gandaglia G, Suardi N, Gallina A, et al. Preoperative erectile function represents a significant predictor of postoperative urinary continence recovery in patients treated with bilateral nerve sparing radical prostatectomy. The Journal of Urology. 2012;**187**:569-574

[89] Klotz L, Heaton J, Jewett M, et al. A randomized phase 3 study of intraoperative cavernous nerve stimulation with penile tumescence monitoring to improve nerve sparing during radical prostatectomy. The Journal of Urology. 2000;**164**(5):1573-1578

[90] Walsh PC, Marschke P, Catalona WJ, et al. Efficacy of first-generation Cavermap to verify location and function of cavernous nerves during radical prostatectomy: A multi-institutional evaluation by experienced surgeons. Urology. 2001;**57**(3):491-494

[91] Kowalcyzk KJ, Huang AC, Hevelone ND, et al. Stepwise approach for nerve sparing without countertraction during robot-assisted radical prostatectomy: Technique and outcomes. European Urology. 2011;**60**:536-547

[92] Sanda MG, Dunn R, Wei J. Seminal vesicle sparing technique is associated with improved sexual HRQOL outcome after radical prostatectomy. The Journal of Urology. 2002;**167**:151

[93] John H, Hauri D. Seminal vesicle sparing radical prostatectomy: A novel concept to restore early urinary continence. Urology. 2000;**55**:820

[94] Gilbert SM, Dunn RL, Miller DC, et al. Functional outcomes following nerve sparing prostatectomy augmented with seminal vesicle sparing compared to standard nerve sparing prostatectomy: Results from a randomized controlled trial. The Journal of Urology. 2017;**198**:600-607

[95] Finley DS, Osann K, Chang A, et al. Hypothermic robotic radical prostatectomy: Impact on continence. Journal of Endourology. 2009;**23**:1443-1450

[96] Finley DS, Chang A, Morales B, et al. Impact of regional hypothermia on urinary continence and potency after robot-assisted radical prostatectomy. Journal of Endourology. 2010;**24**(7):1111-1116

[97] Chien GW, Mikhail AA, Orvieto MA, et al. Modified clipless antegrade nerve preservation in robotic-assisted laparoscopic radical prostatectomy with validated sexual function evaluation. Urology. 2005;**66**:419-423

[98] Eichelberg C, Erbersdobler A, Haese A, et al. Frozen section for the management of intraoperatively detected palpable tumor lesions during nerve-sparing scheduled radical prostatectomy. European Urology. 2006;**49**(6):1011-1018

[99] Schlomm T, Tennstedt P, Huxhold C, et al. Neurovascular structure-adjacent frozen-section examination (NeuroSAFE) increases nerve-sparing frequency and reduces positive surgical margins in open and robot-assisted laparoscopic radical prostatectomy: Experience after 11,069 consecutive patients. European Urology. 2012;**62**(2):333-340

[100] Beyer B, Schlomm T, Tennstedt P, et al. A feasible and time-efficient adaption of NeuroSAFE for da Vinci robot-assisted radical prostatectomy. European Urology. 2014;**66**(1):138-144

[101] Becker A, Coelius C, Adam M, et al. Safe-R. A novel score, accounting for oncological safe nerve-sparing at radical prostatectomy for localized prostate cancer. World Journal of Urology. 2015;**33**(1):77-83

[102] Tewari A, Srivasatava A, Menon M, et al. A prospective comparison of radical retropubic and robot-assisted prostatectomy: Experience in one institution. BJU International. 2003;**92**(3):205-210

[103] Yaxley JW, Coughlin GD, Chambers SK, et al. Robot-assisted laparoscopic prostatectomy versus open radical retropubic prostatectomy: Early outcomes from a randomized controlled phase 3 study. Lancet. 2016;**388**(10049):1057-1066

[104] Sooriakumaran P, Srivastava A, Shariat SF, et al. A multinational, multi-institutional study comparing positive surgical margin rates among 22393 open, laparoscopic, and robot-assisted radical prostatectomy patients. European Urology. 2014;**66**(3):450-456

[105] Novara G, Ficarra V, Mocellin S, et al. Systematic review and meta-analysis of studies reporting oncologic outcome after robot-assisted radical prostatectomy. European Urology. 2012;**62**(3):382-404

[106] Coughlin G, Dangle PP, Palmer KJ, et al. Athermal early retrograde release of the neurovascular bundle during nerve-sparing robotic-assisted laparoscopic radical prostatectomy. Journal of Robotic Surgery. 2009;**3**:13-17

[107] Ko YH, Coelho RF, Sivaraman A, et al. Retrograde versus antegrade nerve sparing during robot-assisted radical prostatectomy: Which is better for achieving early functional recovery? European Urology. 2013;**63**:169-177

[108] Brown JA, Rodin D, Lee B, et al. Transperitoneal versus extraperitoneal approach to laparoscopic radical prostatectomy: An assessment of 156 cases. Urology. 2005;**65**(2):320-324

[109] Phinthusophon K, Nualyong C, Srinualnad S, et al. Laparoscopic radical prostatectomy: Transperitoneal laparoscopic radical prostatectomy versus extraperitoneal endoscopic radical prostatectomy. Journal of the Medical Association of Thailand. 2007;**90**(12):2644-2650

[110] Montorsi F, Brock G, Lee J, et al. Effect of nightly versus on-demand vardenafil on recovery of erectile function in men following bilateral nerve-sparing radical prostatectomy. European Urology. 2008;**54**:924-931

[111] Mostafa ME, Senbel AM, Mostafa T. Effect of chronic low-dose tadalafil on penile cavernous tissues in diabetic rats. Urology. 2013;**81**:1253-1260

[112] Park K, Ryu KS, Li WJ, et al. Chronic treatment with a type 5 phosphodiesterase inhibitor suppresses apoptosis of corporal smooth muscle by potentiating Akt signaling in a rat model of diabetic erectile dysfunction. European Urology. 2008;**53**:1282-1289

[113] Garcia LA, Hlaing SM, Gutierrez RA, et al. Sildenafil attenuates inflammation and oxidative stress in pelvic ganglia neurons after bilateral cavernosal nerve damage. International Journal of Molecular Sciences. 2014;**15**(10):17204-17220

[114] Colombo F, Cogni M, Deiana G, et al. Vacuum therapy. Archivio Italiano di Urologia e Andrologia. 1992;**64**:267-269

[115] Raina R, Agarwal A, Ausmundson S, et al. Early use of vacuum erection device following radical prostatectomy facilitates early sexual activity and potentially earlier return of erectile function. International Journal of Impotence Research. 2006;**18**:77-81

[116] Turner LA, Althof SE, Levine SB, et al. External vacuum devices in the treatment of erectile dysfunction: A one-year study of sexual and psychosocial impact. Journal of Sex & Marital Therapy. 1991;**17**:81-93

[117] Cookson MS, Nadig PW. Long term results with vacuum construction device. The Journal of Urology. 1993;**149**:290-294

[118] Basal S, Wambi C, Acikel C, et al. Optimal strategy for penile rehabilitation after robot-assisted radical prostatectomy based on preoperative erectile function. BJU International. 2012;**111**:658-665

[119] Kohler TS, Pedro R, Hendlin K, et al. A pilot study on the early use of the vacuum erection device after radical retropubic prostatectomy. BJU International. 2007;**100**(4):858-862

[120] Burnett AL. Phosphodiesterase 5 mechanisms and therapeutic applications. The American Journal of Cardiology. 2005;**96**:29M-31M

[121] Carson CC, Lue TF. Phosphodiesterase type 5 inhibitors for erectile dysfunction. BJU International. 2005;**96**:257-280

[122] Wilke RJ, Glick HA, McCarron TJ, et al. Quality of life effects of alprostadil therapy for erectile dysfunction. The Journal of Urology. 1997;**157**(6):2124-2128

[123] Schwartz EJ, Wong P, Graydon RJ. Sildenafil preserves intracorporeal smooth muscle after radical retropubic prostatectomy. The Journal of Urology. 2004;**171**:771-774

[124] Jo JK, Jong JO, Lee SW, et al. Effect of starting penile rehabilitation with sildenafil immediately after robot-assisted laparoscopic radical prostatectomy on erectile function recovery: A prospective randomized trial. The Journal of Urology. 2018;**199**(6):1600-1606

[125] Hyndman ME, Bivalacqua TJ, Feng Z, et al. Nightly sildenafil use after radical prostatectomy has adverse effects on urinary convalescence: Results from a randomized trial of nightly vs. on-demand dosing regimens. Canadian Urological Association Journal. 2015;**9**(11-12):414-419

[126] Zumbé J, Porst H, Sommer F, et al. Comparable efficacy of once-daily versus on-demand vardenafil in men with mild-to-moderate erectile dysfunction: Findings of the RESTORE study. European Urology; 2008;**54**(1):204-210

[127] Tian D, Wang XY, Zong HT, et al. Efficacy and safety of short- and long-term, regular and on-demand regimens of phosphodiesterase type 5 inhibitors in treating erectile dysfunction after nerve-sparing radical prostatectomy: A systematic review and meta-analysis. Clinical Interventions in Aging; 2017;**12**:405-412

[128] Raina R, Agarwal A, Zaramo CE, et al. Long-term efficacy and compliance of MUSE for erectile dysfunction following radical prostatectomy. SHIM (IIEF-5) analysis. International Journal of Impotence Research. 2005;**17**(1):86-90

[129] Raina R, Rahlajani G, Agarwal A, et al. The early use of transurethral alprostadil after radical prostatectomy potentially facilitates an earlier return of erectile function and successful sexual activity. BJU International. 2007;**100**(6):1317-1321

[130] Chang JI, Lam V, Patel MI. Preoperative pelvic floor muscle exercise and postprostatectomy incontinence: A systematic review and meta-analysis. European Urology. 2016;**69**(3):460-467

[131] Hsu LF, Liao YM, Lai FC, et al. Beneficial effects of biofeedback-assisted pelvic floor muscle training in patients with urinary incontinence after radical prostatectomy: A systematic review and metaanalysis. International Journal of Nursing Studies. 2016; **60**:99-111

[132] Lavoisier P, Proulx J, Courtois F, et al. Relationship between perineal muscle contractions, penile tumescence, and penile rigidity during nocturnal erections. The Journal of Urology. 1988;**139**:176

[133] Matthews VB, Astrom MB, Chan MH, et al. Brain-derived neurotrophic factor is produced by skeletal muscle cells in response to contraction and enhances fat oxidation via activation of AMP-activated protein kinase. Diabetologia. 2009;**52**:1409

[134] Dorey G, Speakman MJ, Feneley RC, et al. Pelvic floor exercises for erectile dysfunction. BJU International. 2005;**96**(4):595-597

[135] Perez FS, Rosa NC, Rocha AF, et al. Effects of biofeedback in preventing urinary incontinence and erectile dysfunction after radical prostatectomy. Frontiers in Oncology. 2018;**8**:1-10

[136] Prota C, Gomes CM, Ribeiro LH, et al. Early postoperative pelvic-floor biofeedback improves erectile function in men undergoing radical prostatectomy: A prospective, randomized, controlled trial. International Journal of Impotence Research. 2012; **24**(5):174-178

[137] Muller A, Tal R, Donohue JF, et al. The effect of hyperbaric oxygen therapy on erectile function recovery in a rat cavernous nerve injury model. The Journal of Sexual Medicine. 2008;**5**:562-570

[138] Thom SR. Hyperbaric oxygen—Its mechanisms and efficacy. Plastic and Reconstructive Surgery, Supplement. 2011;**127**:131S

[139] Chiles KA, Staff I, Johnson-Arbor K, et al. A double-blind randomized trial on the efficacy and safety of hyperbaric oxygenation therapy in the preservation of erectile function after radical prostatectomy. The Journal of Urology. 2018;**199**:805-811

[140] Sezen SF, Hoke A, Burnett AL, Snyder, et al. Immunophilin ligand FK506 is neuroprotective for penile innervation. Nature Medicine. 2001;**7**:1073-1074

[141] Mulhall JP, Muller A, Donohue JF, et al. FK506 and erectile function preservation in the cavernous nerve injury model: Optimal dosing and timing. The Journal of Sexual Medicine. 2008;**5**:1334-1344

[142] Lagoda G, Jin L, Lehrfeld TJ, Liu T, Burnett AL. FK506-binding protein localizations in human penile innervation. BJU International. 2008;**101**:604-609

[143] Rahimian R, Fakhfouri G, Rasouli MR, et al. Effect of pioglitazone on sciatic nerve ischemia/reperfusion injury in rats. Pediatric Neurosurgery. 2009;**45**:126-131

[144] Zhu J, Zhang J, Ji M, et al. The role of peroxisome proliferator-activated receptor and effects of its agonist, pioglitazone, on a rat model of optic nerve crush: PPARγ in retinal neuroprotection. PLoS One. 2013;**8**(7):e68935. DOI: 10.1371/journal.pone.0068935

[145] Aliperti LA, Lasker GF, Hagan SS, et al. Efficacy of pioglitazone on erectile function recovery in a rate model of cavernous nerve injury. Urology. 2014;**84**:1122-1127

[146] Gholamine B, Shafiei M, Motevallian M, et al. Effects of pioglitazone on erectile dysfunction in sildenafil poor-responders: A randomized, controlled study. Journal of Pharmaceutical Sciences. 2008;**11**:22-31

[147] Katz EG, Moustafa AA, Heidenberg D, et al. Pioglitazone enhances survival and regeneration of pelvic ganglion neurons after cavernosal nerve injury. Urology. 2016;**89**:76-82

[148] Liang H, Liang P, Xu Y, et al. DHAM-BMSC matrix promotes axonal regeneration and functional recovery after spinal cord injury in adult rats. Journal of Neurotrauma. 2009;**26**:1745-1757

[149] May F, Vroemen M, Matiasek K, et al. Nerve replacement strategies for cavernous nerves. European Urology. 2005;**48**:372-378

[150] Patel VR, Samavedi S, Bates AS, et al. Dehydrated human amnion/chorion membrane allograft nerve wrap around the prostatic neurovascular bundle accelerates early return to continence and potency following robot-assisted radical prostatectomy: Propensity score-matched analysis. European Urology. 2015;**67**:977-980

[151] Ogaya-Pinies G, Palayapalam-Ganapathi H, Rogers T, et al. Can dehydrated human amnion/chorion membrane accelerate the return to potency after a nerve-sparing robotic-assisted radical prostatectomy? Propensity score-matched analysis. Journal of Robotic Surgery. 2017 [E-pub ahead of print]

[152] Yamashita S, Fujii S, Kamiyama Y, et al. Impact of tissue sealing sheet on erectile dysfunction in a rat model of nerve-sparing radical prostatectomy. The Journal of Sexual Medicine. 2016;**13**:1448-1454

[153] Bochinski D, Lin GT, Nunes L, et al. The effect of neural embryonic stem cell therapy in a rat model of cavernosal nerve injury. BJU International. 2004;**94**:904-909

[154] Al-Chalabi A, Miller CC. Neurofilaments and neurological disease. BioEssays. 2003;**25**:346-355

[155] Piao S, Kim IG, Lee JY, et al. Therapeutic effect of adipose-derived stem cells and BDNF-immobilized PLGA membrane in a rat model of cavernous nerve injury. The Journal of Sexual Medicine. 2012;**9**:1968-1979

[156] Jeong HH, Piao S, Ha JN, et al. Combined therapeutic effect of udenafil and adipose-derived stem cell (ASDC)/brain-derived neurotrophic factor (BDNF)-membrane system in a rat model of cavernous nerve injury. Urology. 2013;**81**:1108.e7-1108.e14

[157] Martinez-Salamanca JI, Zurita M, Costa C, et al. Dual strategy with oral phosphodiesterase type 5 inhibition and intracavernosal implantation of mesenchymal stem cells is

superior to individual approaches in the recovery of erectile and cavernosal functions after cavernous nerve injury in rats. The Journal of Sexual Medicine. 2016;**13**(1):1-11

[158] Lin G, Qiu X, Fandel T, et al. Tracking intracavernously injected adipose-derived stem cells to bone marrow. International Journal of Impotence Research. 2011;**23**:268-275

[159] Shan H, Chen F, Zhang T, et al. Stem cell therapy for erectile dysfunction of cavernous nerve injury rats: A systematic review and meta-analysis. PLoS One;**10**(4):e0121428. DOI: 10.1371/journal.pone.0121428

[160] Hou QH, Ge MY, Zhang CD, et al. Adipose tissue-derived stem cell therapy for erectile dysfunction in rats: A systematic review and meta-analysis. International Urology and Nephrology. 2017;**49**(7):1127-1137

[161] Carson 3rd CC. Efficacy of antibiotic impregnation of inflatable penile prostheses in decreasing infection in original implants. The Journal of Urology. 2044;**171**:1611-1614

[162] Garber BB, Marcus SM. Does surgical approach affect the incidence of inflatable penile prosthesis infection? Urology. 1998;**52**:291-293

[163] Eid JF. Penile implant: Review of a "no-touch" technique. Sexual Medicine Reviews. 2016;**4**(3):294-300

[164] Montague DK. Penile prosthesis implantation for end-stage erectile dysfunction after radical prostatectomy. Revista de Urología. 2005;**7**(Suppl 2):S51-S57

[165] Wilson SK, Delk JR, Salem EA, Cleves MA. Long-term survival of inflatable penile prostheses: Single surgical group experience with 2384 first-time implants spanning two decades. The Journal of Sexual Medicine. 2007;**4**:1074-1079

[166] Stember DS, Garber BB, Perito PE. Outcomes of abdominal wall reservoir placement in inflatable penile prosthesis implantation: A safe and efficacious alternative to the space of Retzius. The Journal of Sexual Medicine. 2014;**11**(2):605-612

[167] Ziegelmann MJ, Viers BR, Lomas DJ, Westerman ME, Trost LW. Ectopic penile prosthesis reservoir placement: An anatomic cadaver model of the high submuscular technique. The Journal of Sexual Medicine. 2016;**13**(9):1425-1431

[168] Pillay B, Moon D, Love C, et al. Quality of life, psychosocial functioning, and treatment satisfaction of men who have undergone penile prosthesis surgery following robot-assisted radical prostatectomy. The Journal of Sexual Medicine. 2017;**14**:1612-1620

[169] Megas G, Papadopoulos G, Stathouros G, et al. Comparison of efficacy and satisfaction profile, between penile prosthesis implantation and oral PDE5 inhibitor tadalafil therapy, in men with nerve-sparing radical prostatectomy erectile dysfunction. BJU International. 2013;**112**:E169-E176

[170] Rajpurkar A, Dhabuwala CB. Comparison of satisfaction rates and erectile function in patients treated with sildenafil intracavernous prostaglandin E1 and penile implant surgery for erectile dysfunction in urology practice. The Journal of Urology. 2003;**170**:159-163

[171] Padma-Nathan H, McCullough AR, Levine LA, et al. Randomized, double-blind, placebo-controlled study of postoperative nightly sildenafil citrate for the prevention of erectile dysfunction after bilateral nerve-sparing radical prostatectomy. International Journal of Impotence Research. 2008;**20**:479-486

[172] Pavlovich CP, Levinson AW, Su LM, et al. Nightly vs on-demand sildenafil for penile rehabilitation after minimally invasive nerve-sparing radical prostatectomy: Results of a randomized double-blind trial with placebo. BJU International. 2013;**112**:844-851

[173] Montorsi F, Brock G, Stolzenburg JU, et al. Effects of tadalafil treatment on erectile function recovery following bilateral nerve-sparing radical prostatectomy: A randomized placebo-controlled study (REACTT). European Urology. 2014;**65**:587-596

[174] Canat L, Bayram G, Gurbuz C, et al. Effects of three-times-per-week versus on-demand tadalafil treatment on erectile function and continence recovery following bilateral nerve sparing radical prostatectomy: Results of a prospective, randomized, and single-center study. The Kaohsiung Journal of Medical Sciences. 2015;**31**:90-95

[175] Kim DJ, Hawksworth DJ, Hurwitz LM, et al. A prospective, randomized, placebo-controlled trial of on-demand vs. nightly sildenafil citrate as assessed by RigiScan and the international index of erectile function. Andrology. 2016;**4**:27-32